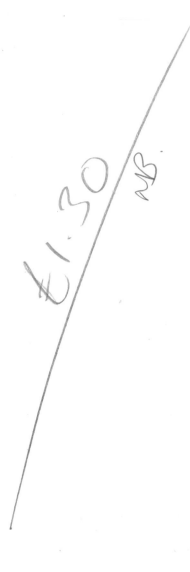

OVERCOMING
ARTHRITIS

Dr Dudley Hart is a general physician who has been actively involved in the field of clinical rheumatism and research into the rheumatic disorders and their treatment. He has contributed to many medical textbooks and publications including those produced by the Arthritis and Rheumatism Council. He has also been involved in clinical trials of many new anti-rheumatic drugs which have now become universally popular. He was for many years consultant at the Westminster Hospital in London and travels widely all over the world lecturing on arthritis and rheumatism.

He has edited a number of books, including *French's Index on Differential Diagnosis, Drug Treatment of the Rheumatic Diseases* and *Joint Disease*.

In his spare time he enjoys caravan holidays and making multi-track musical recordings.

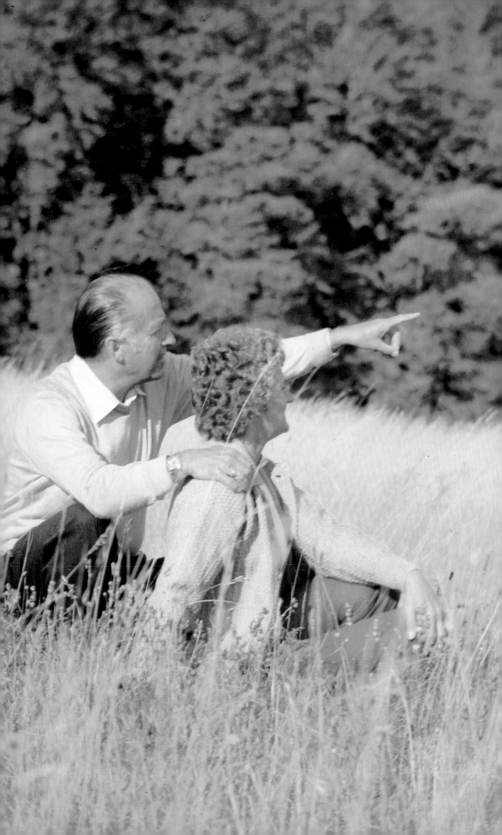

OVERCOMING ARTHRITIS

A guide to coping with stiff or aching joints

Frank Dudley Hart
MD, FRCP

MARTIN DUNITZ

First published in the United Kingdom
in 1981 by Martin Dunitz Ltd.
154 Camden High Street,
London NW1 0NE

**British Library Cataloguing in
Publication Data**
Hart, Francis Dudley
Overcoming arthritis. – (Positive health guides).
1. Arthritis
2. Joints – Diseases
I. Title   II. Series
616-7'2   RC933

ISBN 0-906348-15-3
ISBN 0-906348-13-7 Pbk

Studio photography by Bill Ling

Printed by Toppan Printing Company (S) Pte Ltd, Singapore

CONTENTS

To all the very many arthritic sufferers I
have known who have only rarely
complained, but have got on with the job
of living their lives as best they could to
great effect.

INTRODUCTION

Arthritis and rheumatism are very general terms, covering a wide variety of aches and pains which, taken altogether, probably affect most of us one way or another during our lives. They can include any trouble with the joints from a painful shoulder to a long term illness such as rheumatoid arthritis. Indeed, many people do not realize just what a huge and complex subject arthritis is. This book is intended to be a practical, straightforward guide for any men and women who have aches and pains in their joints and want to know more about what is wrong and if there is anything they can do to relieve the pain and make their daily lives a little easier.

Understanding something about what is happening in your body is the crucial first step towards knowing how best to look after it. I start the book, therefore, with a brief general explanation of how your joints work and what can go wrong with them. Arthritis is not just a single problem of inflammation or deterioration around the bones. It can take a number of entirely different forms. Chapters two and three give a broad survey of the commonest types and the particular differences in approach each one needs.

Many myths have arisen about arthritis. Often the cause of the disease is vague or uncertain and some types can suddenly disappear, either temporarily or forever, for no apparent reason. Both these facts make it a fertile field for speculation and superstition. It is as well to know how many of these beliefs are founded on medically accepted truth and how many are still highly controversial or mere old wives' tales, and the most widespread of them are discussed in chapter four.

Different people find different treatments effective for arthritis, and this is something that can only be decided on with the specific advice of your own doctor who can gear your treatment to suit your individual needs. All that a book like this can do is to give a simple outline of some of the most commonly used forms of relief for arthritic pain and leave you, with your doctor's guidance, to find the right balance according to the nature and severity of your own condition.

Finally there is a section devoted to the wealth of ideas and gadgets that have been devised over the years to help with all the simple, everyday tasks that become suddenly much more difficult when your joints are stiff or painful. It is often amazing how much difference even a small adjustment, such as raising the height of your favourite chair or putting a piece of thickening around your pen, can make to the comfort of your daily activities.

There are as yet no miracle cures for arthritis. But the message is still one of hope and encouragement. Over the years I have met many people who have found ways of learning to live with the pain in their joints and of minimizing the problems and limitations of their disability. This has helped reinforce my conviction that, while many of the difficulties of arthritis cannot be done away with altogether, they can at least, if approached in the right way, be overcome to a heartening and admirable extent.

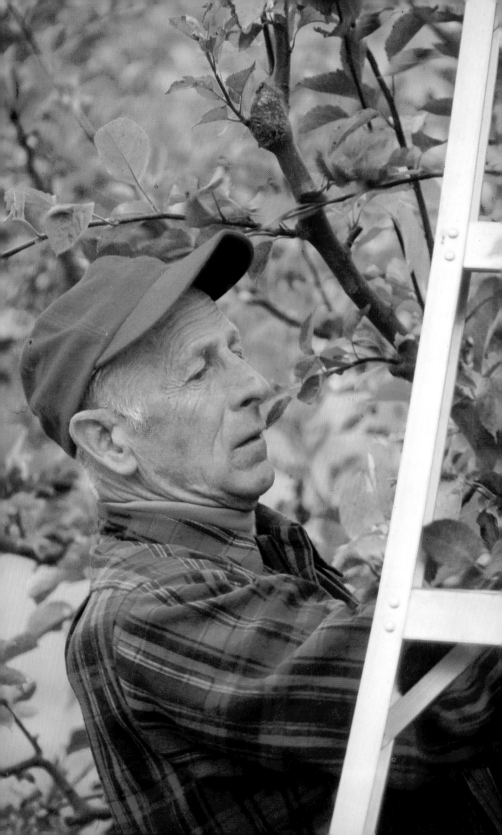

1. WHAT IS ARTHRITIS?

There is a good deal of folklore still present in people's thinking about the rheumatic disorders. Rheumatism as such is a very general term and can refer to any kind of pain in the muscles, bones and joints for which there is no ready explanation. Arthritis is specifically a condition affecting the joints. Strictly speaking the word arthritis should only be used to describe an inflammatory disease and the word arthrosis to describe a condition where the joints are gradually deteriorating. However most forms of arthritis are a mixture of both.

The different kinds

The man in the street does not often realize how many varieties of arthritis there are. In fact there are over 180, each with different causes and different manifestations, and it is obviously essential to get the diagnosis right before deciding on treatment. A rough classification of all the many different kinds of arthritis can be made like this:

1. **Wear and tear** or mainly degenerative (such as osteo-arthrosis). This is when the cartilage inside the joint gradually deteriorates over a period of time, and the bones around it thicken and grow stiff. There will also be a certain amount of inflammation.

2. **Inflammatory** (such as rheumatoid arthritis). The cause of this is not known. The disease may well be started by some infection which causes the joints to become inflamed, but from then on it almost seems as though the body's tissues and defence mechanisms react against themselves and so perpetuate the inflammatory process.

3. **Caused by defects in body chemistry** (such as gout). This sort of inflammation usually only affects one or two joints. In gout the body has too much uric acid and crystals form in the tissues of the joint, producing very intense pain.

4. **Other kinds**. Many arthritic diseases are a mixture of both wear and tear and inflammatory changes. There are also some which are caused by infection, either when the bacteria themselves are taken to the joint

13

(causing septic arthritis), or when the arthritic symptoms occur some time after the infection (as in the case of rheumatic fever and Reiter's/ Brodie's disease). In this second type it seems as though the infection, which may be anything from a sore throat to dysentery can indirectly trigger off changes in the joints though no bacteria are actually transferred there through the blood stream. Septic arthritis can also develop without any earlier symptoms of disease.

5. **Soft tissue rheumatism**: This is where tissues around the joint are affected by injuries, sprains, strains etc and as a result degenerate or become inflamed. Examples would be fibrositis, tennis elbow and similar troubles.

The commonest form is osteo-arthrosis, which most of us are likely to develop to some degree if we live long enough. The more serious rheumatoid arthritis is happily a great deal rarer. The diagram on page 16 shows the relative frequency of various kinds of arthritis.

Each type of arthritis requires a different approach and before you embark on any home treatment it is essential to know which condition you are suffering from. They are discussed individually in the next chapter.

The different sorts are not inter-related, and if you have one kind of arthritis it does not mean that you will get any of the others, although most forms may eventually, if they go on for long enough, lead to 'wear and tear' changes – or in other words to osteo-arthrosis. Aging itself produces these changes as day by day more minor injuries are inflicted on our tissues, but there is a great difference in people's reactions to such insults. Some people's bones and joints are old at forty, some are excellent at seventy. All of us eventually get some features of osteo-arthrosis, but usually not severely. In some ways it is almost a reward for going on living and growing older.

How joints work

Before you can have a proper idea of what arthritis means it is necessary to know something of the nature and structure of a joint. This will vary depending on what the particular joint has to do. Some have to be highly mobile, with a great range of fine movement, as in the case of shoulders and hands. Others, such as hips and knees, have to bear a considerable amount of weight and so have to be essentially stable as well as mobile.

The hand
Put your left hand on your knee and look at the joints of the middle finger

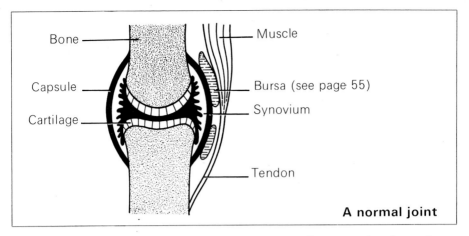

Bone

Capsule

Cartilage

Muscle

Bursa (see page 55)

Synovium

Tendon

A normal joint

as a supreme example of a highly mobile joint. Between the three short bones (or phalanges) in that finger lie the two interphalangeal joints. Each bone is tipped by a soft cushion of cartilage and the space between is moist with synovial fluid. The lining of the joint, or synovium, is surrounded by a capsule or joint sheath in which are many nerve endings.

Normally when you pinch the middle joint of one finger between the finger and thumb of your other hand, either from the sides or from the back and front, you feel pressure but no pain. If the joint becomes inflamed, however, it becomes tender to the pinch, particularly on the sides, and if fluid forms in the joint it becomes swollen, stiff and painful to move. Likewise you can normally make a tight fist and leave the marks of four nails in your palm, or flex the thumb across your palm and wrap your

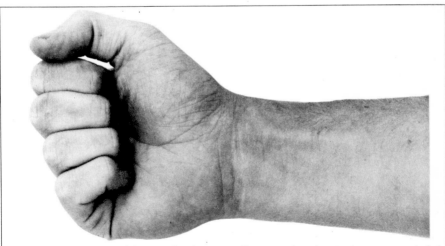

Clenching your hand into a fist is normally easy, but it can become painful or even impossible if you have arthritic fingers.

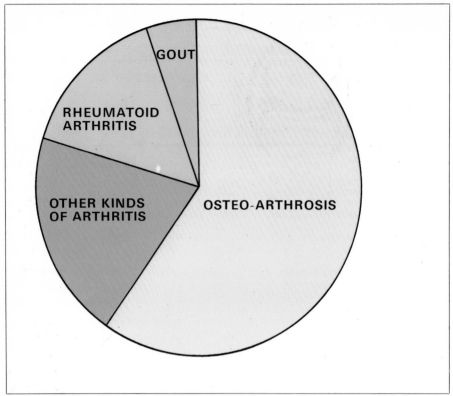

A general comparison of how common different sorts of arthritis are. (Taken from the number of people going to their doctors with arthritic complaints during the course of one year.)

fingers over the top of it with only mild or no discomfort, but as soon as the joints become inflamed these movements can become painful or even impossible to make.

The flexor tendons which bend your fingers into the palm when you make a fist can be felt with the fingers of your other hand but are not easily visible. The extensor tendons running from the wrist over the back of the hand into the fingers can be seen and felt easily. These tendons, which move the fingers into the palm and back again, are surrounded for most of their course to the finger tips by tendon sheaths. At the wrist the tendons run through tunnels up into the arm where they join the main muscles of the forearm. Inside the hand itself are groups of small muscles which work in the hand alone and form the muscular swelling at the base of the thumb on one side and the little finger on the other. Movements of most joints are made by three muscle groups – two opposing each other (for instance the flexors making a fist and the extensors straightening the fingers), and a

16

third stabilizing group which helps maintain intermediate positions.

The hand is a particularly complicated structure in terms of joints, as each finger has three joints and the thumb two. At the wrist, movements occur between the two bones of the forearm and the small bones of the wrist, where the eight carpal bones move like two rows of pebbles packed on one another.

The fine movements which made man what he is today and enable him to perform his very refined actions depend on the smooth interaction of these fifteen joints in each hand plus the more restricted movements between the carpal bones. Some joints, like those at the middle and end of each finger, move in two directions only (to and fro, as it were), but in the knuckle joints sideways movements are also possible and the wrist can make both these and rotatory movements.

The arm

At the elbow there are two separate joints, one the forearm on the arm bone (which can move up and down or to and fro), and the other a rotatory movement between the two bones of the forearm which enables us to turn our palms upwards or downwards (which means, for example, that we can read the time on our wristwatches whether we wear them on the back or the front of our wrist).

The shoulder

The shoulder joint is even more subtle and really consists of three separate joints:

1. Movement of the arm bone (humerus) on the shoulder blade.

2. Movement of the shoulder blade on the ribs.

3. Movement of the collar bone or clavicle on the shoulder blade.

The subtle art of the tennis player when he is serving the ball brings in not just these three shoulder movements but both of the elbow and

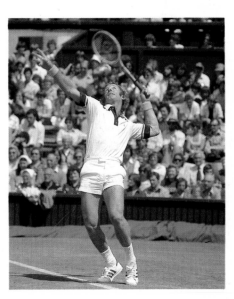

The co-ordination of many different joint movements is needed to carry out a powerful and well executed service.

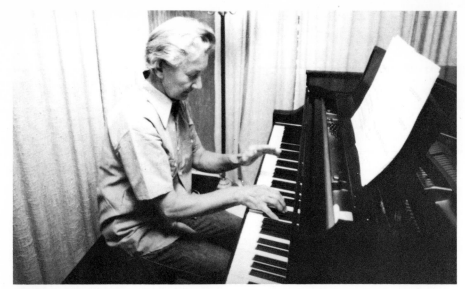

Precise, complex movements such as those a pianist has to make with his fingers are generally the worst affected by even a small amount of damage to the joints.

most of the hand movements also. When any of the joints performing such fine movements are upset by injury or arthritis it is no great wonder that function suffers greatly and fine movements suffer most. A hand seriously affected by arthritis can still usually write or type letters and perform tasks of no great complexity but the pianist, for instance, cannot any longer play competently as his art depends on full, fluid movement of all the components of his joints.

The hip

Joints of the upper half of the body, such as the arm, have to be mobile and capable of fine movements, but the leg joints also have to carry the body's weight around, and are constructed accordingly. The hip, for instance, is a ball and socket joint with the head of the thigh bone (femur) deeply placed in a cup-shaped hollow at the side of the pelvis. Movements here have to be fluid and supple but, at the same time, the joint is a very solid one so that it can carry the weight of the body straight down onto the femur below. It is surrounded by some of the strongest muscles in the body and is able to move in a multitude of different directions.

The knee

The main movements in the knee are flexion and extension (forwards and backwards). This, however, is accompanied when walking by a slight sliding forwards of bone on bone which makes it rather more subtle than just a simple hinge movement. The patella or knee cap over the front of the knee is merely a large bony island in the muscle tendon.

The ankle and foot

Unlike the knee, the ankle is capable not only of forwards and backwards but also of rotatory movements, rather like a modified version of the wrist. But, alas, our poor toes are now nothing like as supple as our fingers and are capable of relatively little individual movement. In fact they are not particularly useful to us any more, although the big toe does a great deal of work and is the joint, above all others, that gets injured by repeated movements and, even more commonly, by the wearing of unsuitable shoes. There is relatively little movement between the individual joints of the toes. This is because we have ceased to use them as fingers and no longer swing through the branches of the trees. The rest of the foot, however, remains supple, especially among people who spend some of the time walking barefoot. In countries where the people do not wear shoes all the time as a matter of course, their feet remain remarkably flexible.

The spine

The bones of the spine are a much more complicated affair. Not only does each vertebra move on the one below it through a piece of cartilage or disc, but there is also, at the back of the spine, a joint between each one.

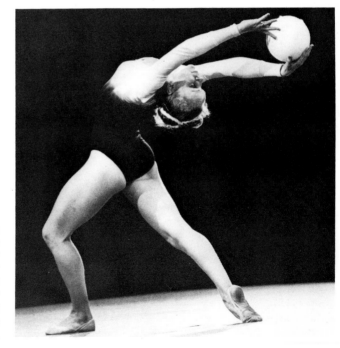

Not all of us can move our spines as spectacularly as this, but our backs are capable of a wider variety of movements than many people realize.

The spinal cord runs through a channel in these vertebrae and the various nerves come out through small holes called foramina. The spine therefore has to be very stable as it protects this vital nervous tissue which, if damaged, would cause paralysis. At the same time it has to be quite mobile. The movements are mainly flexion and extension, i.e. forwards and backwards, but the back can also be moved sideways and turned to the left and right by rotatory movements. As we grow older these movements become more restricted, but there is also a great difference between individuals, and even at eighteen years old some youths are much more supple than others.

What can go wrong with a joint

What happens when a joint is stricken by injury or disease? The simplest example is a strain, as in an ankle injury caused by a wrench or a twist. The joint becomes swollen with fluid, the blood supply to the part increases and it becomes warm and painful. Movement is restricted because of swelling and pain, and the sufferer avoids putting weight on the affected joint and rests it. If you fracture a bone, even if pain is not severe you can usually feel instinctively that you should avoid putting weight on it. Something tells you all is not right in the affected area. A strain or wrench usually gets better in a few days or weeks though a fractured bone takes a month or more to heal. Inflammation of this kind can also be caused by disease, as for example in gout, which likewise usually gets better quite quickly.

After injury or an attack of gout there is an obvious cause for the joint becoming inflamed, but in rheumatoid arthritis there is no such obvious reason, and the disease itself appears to be the source of the inflammation.

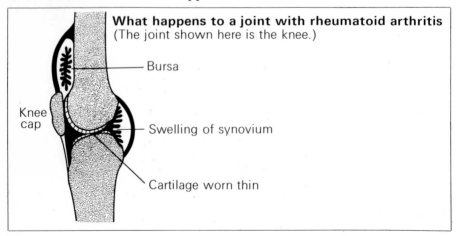

What happens to a joint with rheumatoid arthritis
(The joint shown here is the knee.)

Bursa

Knee cap

Swelling of synovium

Cartilage worn thin

Where this progresses unchecked the joint can become distorted as the cartilage gradually gets destroyed and the ligaments loosen. The function of the joint becomes impaired, causing deformities, stiffness or, occasionally, unnatural mobility. Once the smooth harmonic balance between different bones and muscles has been harmed, the joint ceases to work efficiently and the muscles serving it become weaker. This has a most depressing effect, especially if the working of the joint becomes so severely restricted as to prevent the poor sufferer from leading a normal life.

In osteo-arthrosis there is relatively little inflammation and the problem is rather different. What happens here is that the cartilages, or the soft cushions between the bones, start to lose their elasticity as they age. They become friable and the bones each side also start to change, often thickening in texture and throwing out bony lumps, so that although the parts may be more sturdy and stronger than before, the joints start to grow stiff, and hurt if they are moved.

Injury or inflammation may cause a big increase in the amount of fluid in a joint, so that it may start to bulge – water on the knee is an example of this. Joint fluid is not a secretion from the glands, but a natural fluid from the circulation which increases when there is any inflammation or irritation in the joint.

Early signs of arthritis

We all get occasional aches and pains in the joints and it is not always easy to tell the cause or to know which pains matter and which don't. It is possible to get very hypochondriacal and imagine, quite wrongly, that every minor inexplicable ache is a sign of the onset of arthritis. As a

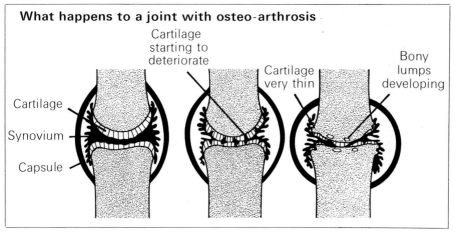

What happens to a joint with osteo-arthrosis

Cartilage starting to deteriorate

Cartilage very thin

Bony lumps developing

Cartilage

Synovium

Capsule

general rule pains that don't last long, such as an occasional prickling or stabbing, probably don't mean anything, but if you get longer periods of pain, swelling, stiffness and weakness in your joints then you should have it checked by your family doctor.

The different kinds of arthritis have different symptoms and are described separately in chapter two. However what most people are worried about when they first get joint pains is whether they might be a sign of osteo- or rheumatoid arthritis and a few simple and reasonably reliable general facts can help distinguish between these two.

Osteo-arthrosis usually only affects people over the age of fifty and takes the form of a persistent, dull ache or burning in some of the joints which gradually grow stiff and knobbly and more difficult to move. The toes, knees, hips, hands and neck are most likely to be affected and will often ache worse after exercise, getting less painful when they are rested.

Rheumatoid arthritis, which is much rarer, can affect any age group. The pain often starts in the knuckles or bases of the toes. The hands may swell up and become puffy, stiff and tender to the touch. If it starts with the fingers it tends to afflict the first joint, as opposed to osteo-arthrosis which affects the end joint. There may also be stiffness or pain on moving the shoulders, knees, hips or elbows. Rheumatoid arthritis nearly always affects both sides of the body at once, and not just one hand or hip (as may be the case in osteo-arthrosis). It is often worse after rest and particularly bad in the early morning, and it doesn't just make for painful joints but also gives the patient a general sense of being ill and run down.

In the majority of cases the onset of either osteo-arthrosis or rheumatoid arthritis is gradual although about one in ten instances of rheumatoid arthritis start abruptly and osteo-arthrosis may sometimes appear to come on suddenly after a joint has been injured in an accident. Fuller details on both these and other kinds of arthritis are given in the next chapter.

2. WHAT ARE THE DIFFERENT TYPES?

Osteo-arthrosis

Osteo-arthrosis is common not only to all mankind, but to every vertebrate animal. All animals with bones and cartilages suffer some degenerative changes in them if they live long enough, but this aging process varies immensely depending on one's forebears, how much injury the joint has suffered in the past and various other factors. A hip, for instance, is more likely to develop osteo-arthrosis if it has been dislocated or fractured – particularly if it was damaged when being set or returned to its socket.

In a few families osteo-arthrosis sets in in the thirties in several joints, in others the members of the family remain free until they are seventy or eighty. In general, however, almost everybody has some signs of degenerative change by the time they are fifty or sixty years old, at the base of the neck, in the lower spine, the big toes and, to a lesser extent, the knees. But osteo-arthrosis can affect any joint anywhere, particularly if it has previously suffered some injury or disease. A joint which was once operated upon may sometimes be more prone to osteo-arthritic changes later, but this very much depends on the nature of the operation and the excellence of the results.

The general effect of osteo-arthrosis affecting several joints is to slow up the sufferer. Athletic patients resent this extremely and a man who used to be a long distance runner may find he can hardly move without extreme discomfort; a rowing man that his knees and hips are so stiff and painful that he cannot walk any distance, let alone row a boat. All this is very thwarting and bad for the morale and the temper. The rest of the family may note that father (or mother) is not the sweet gentle soul he used to be and that he is becoming more crotchety in his old age. O.A. (old age) is bad enough, grandparents may feel, without having O.A. (osteo-arthrosis) in addition.

Generalized osteo-arthrosis

This variety of arthrosis affects many more women than men and commonly occurs at or soon after the menopause or 'change of life'. It usually starts with soreness and pricking in the end joints of the fingers and often also in the bases of the thumbs near the wrist. The parts become

23

gradually thickened and sometimes quite acutely tender with little cysts at the end of the finger which disappear and settle within a year. What starts as a pricking or an initial discomfort soon settles down and the ends of the fingers and the thumb bases are left somewhat thick and knobbly ('granny's hand') but relatively or completely painless. At the shoulder it is the joint at the end of the clavicle or collar bone and not the true shoulder joint that is likely to be affected.

It sometimes runs in families, grandmother passing on the tendency to mother, who in turn passes it on to her child. It is a nuisance disease rather than a serious one. It does not affect your general health or your insurance policies, but it does cause discomfort and pain and can be a considerable annoyance to the sufferer. Men also get a similar arthritis but much less often and later in life.

It seems as though the disorder is due to a mixture of genetic and hormonal factors. It tends to appear as the female hormones are diminishing in the body and it is aggravated by repeated minor injuries, the joints which it affects in the fingers and toes being those most vulnerable to frequent mild knocks. For this reason the joint at the end of the right index finger is often the first to be affected in right-handed people, and the left in left-handed people. The big toes are very often adversely affected by ill-fitting shoes which are too tight and compress the big toe or pull it sideways over the others.

Similar degenerative changes in the discs and joints of the spine are responsible for diseases in the lower spine particularly if it has once been injured. These back troubles will be discussed later.

Types of pain and how to ease them
Pain in any of the rheumatic conditions is what the disease is all about. Pain takes you to your doctor and it is pain-relieving medicines that are perhaps the most helpful of all the drugs used in the treatment of osteo-arthrosis. However, much can be done to control and prevent pain without resorting to the medicine bottle.

Let us take the knee as an example. Sitting with the knee in a fixed position, as for instance when you are watching television for periods of more than thirty minutes at a time, will very often cause aggravation of the pain in and around the knee cap. The ache becomes so bad that eventually you will have to get out of your chair, rub your knees, stretch your legs and walk about a little. The same problem commonly arises in theatres (less so in cinemas where the seats are usually more comfortable and

Shopping expeditions can be very hard on arthritic knees. Taking regular rests, preferably with your legs out as straight as you comfortably can, is one way to make the ordeal less painful.

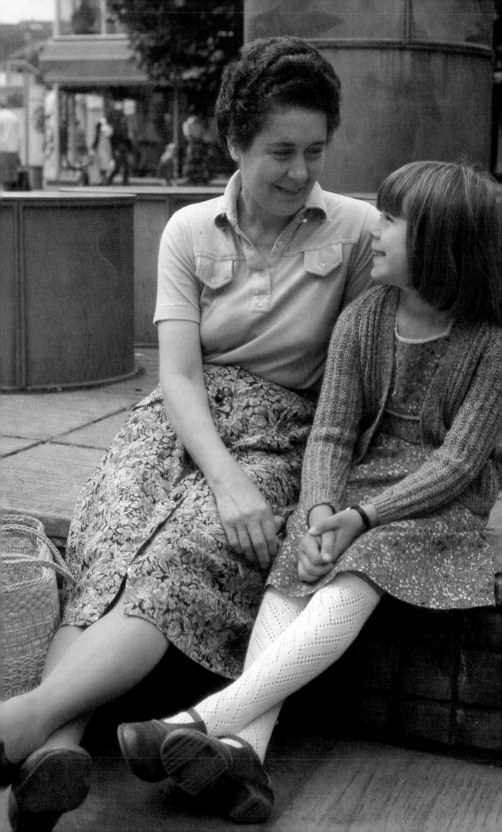

spacious) and in seats in aircraft where there is very often far too little room for your knees unless you are a midget! This pain from immobility is a nuisance while it lasts but is soon cured by movement, simple massage and straightening your legs.

The second type of pain is entirely different. It arises from prolonged standing or exercise – that is, from weight-bearing, walking on hard surfaces or going on long shopping expeditions – an activity guaranteed to aggravate osteo-arthrosis in the knees. The general rule is not to persist for more than an hour at a time without having a rest, taking the weight off your legs and if possible resting your knees straight rather than bent, although this is sometimes difficult to do outside your own home. This kind of pain applies to all joints that carry the weight of the body, and particularly to the knees.

A third pain of osteo-arthrosis is caused by the stretching of the tissues when you make full or exaggerated movements. A tight bending of the knee for instance may cause great pain, and going up, or more particularly down stairs can be a very unpleasant experience as the joint is then under considerable stress. Bending the legs while your weight is on them, as when you squat down to brush mats or empty low drawers, raises the pressure inside knees considerably and aggravates pains, so any prolonged squatting should be avoided. Of all exertions the Russian dance with knees fully bent would undoubtedly have the worst effect on arthritic knees!

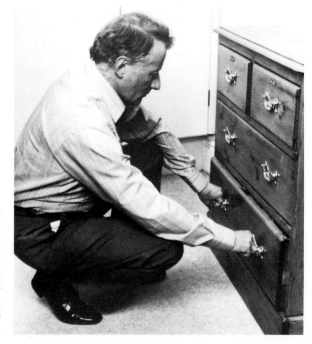

Bending your joints tightly, especially when all your weight is on them, can be agony. Try to keep anything you find you need regularly in higher drawers to spare yourself unnecessary bending.

Rheumatoid arthritis

This is one of the more unpleasant forms of arthritis. It is an inflammatory condition which affects many joints, particularly those in the hands, arms and legs. It may also occasionally affect the jaws, but does not usually trouble the spine, although it can in severe cases. It is more common in adults than in children but anybody from the age of two to ninety or more can develop the disease. It is three times more common among women than men.

The cause is unknown, and for no apparent reason several or many joints of the body will suddenly become inflamed. It is usually symmetrical, which means that one side of the body is affected much the same as the other. In other words, if you get it in your right wrist, your left wrist will also suffer from it. The joints show some swelling, cannot move properly and are tender when pressure is put on them. A characteristic feature of rheumatoid arthritis is that the joint pains, swelling and stiffness are more marked in the early morning so the unfortunate sufferer feels worse when he wakes up than at any other time of the day. He may be so stiff that he is hardly able to move. However, after half an hour or so of limbering up he will start to feel much better and can move around more easily.

The tell-tale signs early on are:

1. Pain and tenderness in the bases or balls of the toes when walking.

2. Sore, stiff and swollen fingers and wrists.

3. Painful restriction of movement and often considerable swelling in the shoulders, elbows and knees.

The patient not only suffers the effects of pain and disablement but also feels run down and sometimes quite ill as the symptoms may include a slight fever.

The disease may last for several months or for considerably longer. It can switch off completely at any time and one always hopes that it will do so. Unfortunately a number of cases go on for many years, but only a few progress relentlessly to the point of severe crippling. It is quite common for the disease to switch off and then switch on again later and, of course, if we could discover what caused these stops and starts we would be in a much better position to treat the malady.

It is naturally very disabling and depressing and, as one patient said to me, 'Every night is an unpleasant experience and I wake in the morning tired out and worse than when I went to bed.' The fact that it goes on and on is one of the most depressing aspects, as there often seems to be no future and every day is like the last one. However, it is comforting to remember that this disease can switch off, either partly or completely. The fact that nature can produce a cure on occasion makes us all hopeful that the secret of the ailment will be discovered before many more years have gone by.

It is only in a minority of cases that there is more than one rheumatoid arthritic in a family. Although there are a few families where the disease tendency seems to be passed on to one or more of the children, this is quite rare. It is however possible that people with certain antigens in their cells (that is, people who are of a special tissue type) are more liable to develop it than others.

As there is no certain cure, doctors usually speak of management, rather than treatment, of rheumatoid arthritis. This management has to a large extent to be done by the patient, for although there are many drugs available such as pain killers, anti-inflammatory (anti-rheumatic) medicines and medicines that apparently work on the disease process itself at a deeper level, such as gold injections, much of the treatment and its effectiveness depends on the patient's own attitude towards the disorder.

Overcoming the depression

In rheumatoid arthritis patients naturally become very anxious about the future. Will their job still be there for them when they return from hospital or after a period off work? Will they be able to do it? Will the busy housewife be able to do her housework and look after her children satisfactorily? Anxiety is very much a part of rheumatoid arthritis, and often seems particularly acute at night. If you are being kept awake by your illness these can be, in every sense of the words, your darkest hours as all worries loom very large and the future looks doubly bleak. Your doctor can give you medicines to relieve anxiety, but probably the best way to ease it is to 'get it out of your system' by talking about your worries to a sympathetic listener.

Rheumatoid arthritis is a disheartening disease and tends in many cases to produce quite a deep depression for a time. You should try not to allow this to happen if you can avoid it, although it is impossible not to feel down-hearted on occasion. However, if depression takes over and your spirits go down and down then you will tend to do less, to sit around more and to become more stiff, so that in the end things will be made infinitely worse. It is a disease that you must fight mentally as well as (with the brakes on) physically.

Mental depression tends to diminish the effects of the drugs you are taking so that you may begin to find that even the common aspirin does

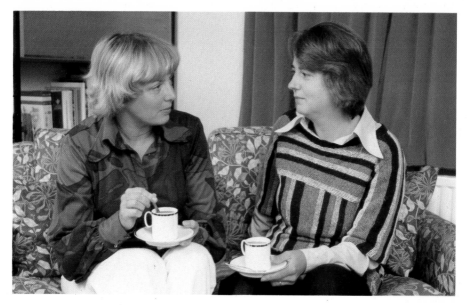

It often helps a lot to be able to talk about your worries to a sympathetic friend rather than to suffer in silence.

not work as well as it did. Happily, your doctor can give you one of quite a large number of medicines which do help depression, and these need not make you dopy or sleepy. However, as with anxiety, the best way to avoid getting depressed is to talk to somebody about your troubles. Even in the busy surgery or clinic you may get the greatest benefit from exchanging ideas and receiving a little understanding.

Patients with sympathetic and helpful families are of course in a much better position than those who are living alone. It is particularly depressing to have to fight a chronic inflammatory disease like rheumatoid arthritis without help. A visiting physician, physiotherapist, nurse, relative or any understanding and sympathetic friend is of particular help for people who live alone as they need to be able to talk about their difficulties and get some practical advice. Neighbours can be helpful in this respect provided that any suggestions they give on treatment are really suitable for you. Quite often people can give advice which is actually intended for some other form of arthritis as they do not realize how many different sorts there are and that not all have the same forms of treatment.

Rest and activity – finding the right balance

Every patient is an individual with different problems and requirements. Some rest is essential in all cases but how much you need will depend entirely on the severity of the condition. If you have very acute

29

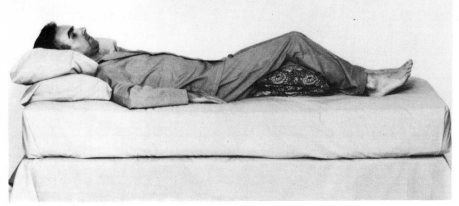

Wrong: Never sleep with your knees resting over a cushion.

rheumatoid arthritis you must rest in bed until the inflamed joints settle down, but you should nonetheless perform simple movements several times a day to exercise every joint in the body and prevent stiffness creeping in. You can do this either in bed or sitting on the side of it.

When resting it is important to be in the correct position. Lying in bed with nothing to support your feet and with the bedclothes tight over them tends to pull the toes down and as a result the ankles may become stiff and the feet dropped and painful. Similarly putting a cushion under your knees can be dangerous for if you sleep with the knees bent over a pillow (which is very comfortable) you may find within a few days or nights that you cannot straighten your knees. It is therefore essential to rest for much of the time with the legs straight. If you spend all day sitting down or lying in bed with bent legs your knees can become permanently fixed in this position. When this happens the hips may also become stiff and bent so when the patient gets out of bed he or she can hardly hobble around as both hips and knees are flexed almost to a right angle.

Rest must also be accompanied by repeated 'de-freezing' exercises so that all the joints of the body are put, as far as possible, through their full range of movement every day. Suggestions on exercises are given in the section on pages 70 to 76. A cage or cradle over the bed holding the bedclothes off the knees and feet is essential to enable you to do some of them.

The more affected joints, of course, cannot go through their full range because of pain, but you should take the movement as far as it will go without hurting, and then back again, and see if the point of pain can be gently extended day by day and week by week.

In conjunction with the daily exercises given in chapter five you may want to try using 'assisted' movement. One example is the following.

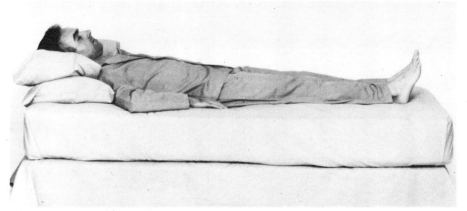

Right: Your joints will benefit if you keep them straight, but not stretched.

Stand facing and fairly close to the wall, running your fingers up the wall in front of you until your hand is as high as possible above the shoulders and then swing your arms slowly sideways with a semi-circular movement down the wall until they are back at your sides. This can be done three or four times a day, with half a dozen movements each time. Even people in normal health may feel some discomfort as the arms approach right angles with the body at shoulder level, and can therefore benefit from these exercises. The elbows should also be extended and bent several times a day, and the wrists flipped up and down and to and fro and around about with circular movements so that the wrists and fingers likewise do not become stiff.

The amount of daily rest can be reduced as soon as acute symptoms have abated, but when you start to get about the house again you should keep periods of rest each morning and afternoon. Quite a good plan is to rest with your feet off the ground for half an hour to an hour every morning and one to two hours every afternoon on a bed or couch. Movements and exercises are best done after a hot bath or shower when the parts are warm and glowing and more mobile.

Clothing and footwear

If your feet, hips and knees (i.e. the weight-bearing joints) are affected, there are certain practical points you should bear in mind. Shoes may become very tight and uncomfortable when feet swell and become arthritic. You should not therefore cram your feet into tight or pointed shoes. It does not matter what they look like, it is how comfortable they are that matters. Wide, soft, flat-heeled shoes which do not press on each side of the toes are essential. Tight socks and stockings which compress the toes should also be avoided and when out of doors in cold weather you

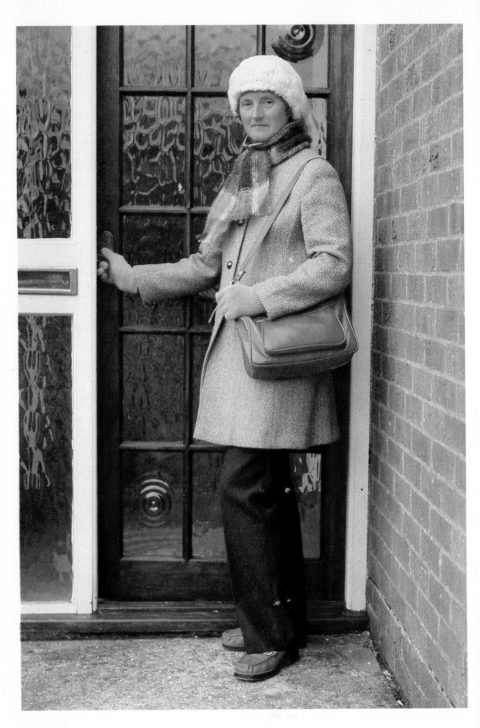

Make sure you are warmly dressed whenever there is a chill in the air.

should wear long warm gloves which cover your wrists. Trousers keep the knees and lower part of the body warmer than skirts and men find 'long johns' (or long underpants) warmer and better than the modern, brief varieties. In other words sensible warm clothing on cold days when in or out of doors is essential because cold and damp, although they do not cause or basically aggravate the disease, do make the aches and pains worse.

Diet

Diet does not make a great deal of difference in rheumatoid arthritis. Vegetarians get the disease and so do meat eaters. Nobody is immune. One of the oldest treatments in the world is starvation, but patients with rheumatoid arthritis have usually lost weight and if anything they need a little more rather than less nutrition. Your diet should therefore be a full normal one to your own liking – not too much and not too little, with enough protein and all the necessary vitamins. If you have had rheumatoid arthritis for a long time the proteins in your blood will tend to be low and your appetite poor, so a full good diet is generally to be encouraged. However, patients who are very much overweight can find this an added nuisance when they are trying to get about again on inflamed and painful joints, and in such cases a slimming diet with restriction of starches and sugar is essential. It is painful enough carrying a normal weight around the house when you have rheumatoid arthritis, and every additional pound or kilo makes life that much more difficult.

Although there are many different types of diet which some patients claim are good for their particular condition, this is an individual decision. Mrs Smith's diet which she finds delightful and which suits her best may not be at all popular with Mrs Brown or Mrs Robinson who each swear by something entirely different. Provided it is sensible, sufficiently nutritious and not too fattening, then any diet which you like and can get on with is the right one.

Some people have indigestion or ulcers, and the combination of rheumatoid arthritis with a duodenal or gastric ulcer is very unpleasant as so many of the medicines that are given for rheumatoid arthritis tend to upset the stomach. In such cases the diet has to be modified in terms of both the indigestion and the ulcer. Strong spicy and fried foods should be kept to a minimum if you find that they upset you. Generally speaking meats, fresh fruits and green vegetables are excellent provided they are not eaten in excessively large amounts.

Many people fear that acid foods and fruit are bad for them if they have rheumatoid arthritis, but this is not so. Simple fruit acids do not affect it as acidity plays no part at all in the disease.

Hand deformities

There is one deformity which is common in rheumatoid arthritis and this is the so-called ulnar deviation, in which the fingers wander away from the thumb towards the little finger which bends sideways. They can always be easily restored by the other hand to their normal position but rebound again as soon as the correcting pressure is removed. Special splints can be worn in bed at night or in the day, but the deformities tend to recur as soon as the splints are removed. The splints may help stabilize the hand and slow up or prevent further deformities occurring. However what matters most with the hand is that you should be able to use it. An ugly looking, somewhat deformed hand that can be used effectively is far better than an elegant looking but less useful one.

Bed sores

In rheumatoid arthritis small nodules may appear over elbows and buttocks and wherever there is pressure on a bone. Care should always be taken to protect these areas, as they can ulcerate, particularly over buttocks, if they are pressed too much on hard surfaces. In bed to prevent sores you can put a lambskin (either synthetic or natural) under your buttocks and hips. Other pressure points are elbows and heels and patients confined to bed for any length of time should take particular care to protect these. You should change position as often as possible or, if you find you have to stay lying or sitting all day, try to get up and move around a bit every hour or so.

Gout

In the old days no distinction was made between different sorts of arthritis and up to around 1880 almost everything was called gout, gouty arthritis or gouty something else. In fact, although gout is quite common, several other forms of arthritis, particularly osteo-arthrosis, are a great deal more so.

Gout has been known and written about for hundreds of years – records go back as far as pre-Christian times. It is a good example of a disease which is very often inherited. The defect lies in the body containing too much urate and uric acid – either because too much is made or because too little is cleared by the kidneys. (There is, incidentally, a popular belief that acid also has a lot to do with many other sorts of arthritis, but this is not true.) What happens is that crystals of monosodium biurate crystallize out in the tissues of a joint and cause intense irritation. All the four basic features of inflammation appear – redness, swelling, pain and dysfunction. Increased blood flow to the area causes intense pain and the redness and swelling cause difficulty in moving and more pain.

Acute gout can hardly be confused with anything else. It is a disease which mainly affects men – in women it is rare at any age and, indeed, almost non-existent before the menopause. The victim of gout is usually (but not always) somewhat overweight, and he is often a healthy, hearty looking person who eats and drinks well and leads a good positive life. He goes to bed fit and well, after having perhaps had a party or indulged in heavy exercise or done something else which was unusual for him. At about 5.00 in the morning he wakes with a most acute pain, usually in the big toe joint, which feels as though he has broken it and, rising out of bed, he finds this joint so tender that he cannot put it on the floor. It is acutely sensitive to the touch, and is red, smarting and swollen. If at 4.00 or 5.00 in the morning you find your big toe has suddenly become transformed into an extremely painful shining tomato of a joint, that is gout. All arthritic conditions are painful, but gout is much more than this and is really an agony. Happily it soon comes under control when adequately treated.

What causes gout

People with this problem nearly always have a high level of uric acid in the blood but they do not generally develop gout until middle age. There are many causes for a high level of uric acid, not all of which are very serious. In men the natural uric acid level in the blood tends to rise at adolescence and in women at the menopause. The level can be raised by overeating and lowered by losing weight. It is often influenced by heredity and if your family has had a tendency towards high uric acid levels you may inherit it.

I have already said that a good party or an excessive amount of exercise or anything that breaks your normal routine may precipitate an attack, but there are two other causes which are quite common today. One is a starvation diet. Starvation makes the uric acid rise in the blood and this may produce an acute attack of gout. So the overweight man rather subject to gout who goes to a health farm and starves himself seriously to lose weight may, in fact, precipitate further attacks. It is just as well, if you wish to reduce your weight and you have gout, to do it gradually and lose a small amount each week because the loss of much more may precipitate an acute attack.

Another common cause for precipitation of an acute attack is the use of diuretics. These are most efficient drugs for getting water out of the system if the body becomes water logged for any reason, such as heart failure, but the brisk output of water caused by a large and efficient dose of one of these diuretics may also precipitate an acute episode of gout.

Treatment

Until recently the only drug that was helpful for gout was colchicine which was derived from the autumn crocus or meadow saffron. This drug did noble work from the time of the Greeks onwards. It is still popular and is in wide use, but can have the side-effect of causing diarrhoea which is sometimes severe. There are also many other drugs for gout which do not have these unpleasant effects and which get the attack under control just as well. Colchicine has 2000 years of usage to its credit, but has now become only one of several treatments available.

Whatever is used in gout has to be used quickly and in full dosage otherwise the condition can drag on and become most unpleasant and very crippling. However with effective early treatment the sufferer can usually walk within twenty-four or forty-eight hours and is back to normal within a week. More than thirty years ago one used to see cases of chronic gout with large deposits of urate showing through the skin, yellowish or white in colour, very often in the ears or around the knuckles or sometimes in the feet or over the elbows. These so-called tophi used to be not uncommon but are now becoming relatively rare and with modern drugs in wide usage will probably disappear completely within the next twenty or thirty years (we hope!).

Prevention

In summary, then, gout is today a preventable disease, and depends on the following things:

1. Not all gout sufferers are overweight but the majority are and a gradual and steady slimming programme is essential.

2. If you have a high uric acid level and your father or grandfather had gout then it is wise to avoid taking excessive amounts of food or alcohol at any one time.

3. Be careful what you eat and in particular avoid foods which are high in uric acid. For instance, fish roes, kidneys, livers and offal of any sort may, in large amounts, precipitate an acute attack. Other foods you should avoid taking in excessive quantities are meat extracts, thick gravies, sweetbreads, hearts, brain, anchovies, sardines, whitebaits, sprats and smelts. Of the alcoholic drinks, the ones most likely to bring on acute gout are heavy beers, port, strong red wine and occasionally champagne. (It is the proud boast of most Scotsmen that gout is rarer in Scotland because they drink whisky.)

4. When you go on holiday always remember to take your drugs with you. Gout is often known as the weekend or holiday disease because it

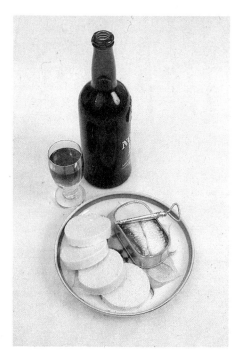

Foods high in uric acid, such as fish roe, sardines or a glass of port can bring on an attack of gout.

usually strikes when you are far from home, and very often at night when the pharmacies or drug stores are shut. If you have your own medicine in your pocket and take it immediately, then the attack usually settles down quite quickly.

5. There are also several long term agents which can be given to lower the uric acid and this means taking one or two tablets every day probably for the rest of your life. But if the pills prevent these agonising episodes it is worth it, for not only do they stop you getting acute gout but they stop the urate collecting in the tissues and return the uric acid in the blood and body to normal levels. However these preventive drugs should only be started on doctor's orders and in periods between attacks. They are not the same as the drugs used to combat acute gout and if taken during an attack may actually worsen or prolong it. But, under your doctor's instructions, you can learn to use the two types of drug correctly in conjunction and so bring the problem of gout under control.

Gout used to be called the Disease of Lords and the Lord of Diseases but nowadays almost everybody can afford it as it does not have to result from a great deal of rich living. However it is also true today that anyone, by obeying the general advice given here, can greatly reduce the chances of being struck by gout.

Other kinds of arthritis

Ankylosing spondylitis

Ankylosing spondylitis is a relatively uncommon disease which mainly affects men. Women can also occasionally get it, but generally in a milder form. In several cases there is a family history of the disease and either the father, mother or another relative is found to have suffered from it.

Sometimes children start with early signs of the illness (such as a swelling in the knee or ankle) when they are at school, but the usual time of onset is between the ages of seventeen and twenty-seven. The first symptom is most often an aching in the buttocks which starts on one side, moving soon to the other side and then settling in both, the discomfort passing down the back of the thighs. It is usually a persistent ache and may be associated early on with swelling in the knees or ankles. Pain and stiffness in the hips and back and a sense of restriction around the ribs are also common. A characteristic symptom is marked stiffness on waking in the morning and the whole spine may be so stiff and painful that the patient has to roll himself out of bed.

One thing which makes ankylosing spondylitis different from other arthritic disorders is its tendency to stiffen the back. After a period of time it can in some cases cause a rigid, so-called 'poker' spine. This was much more common in the old days than it is today, the reason being that in the past patients with the disease were often immobilized, either in bed or in plaster jackets, which was a thoroughly bad thing as it made the stiffening of the spine even worse.

When the diagnosis is made, therefore, it is important to maintain exercise and activities of all sorts. It is helpful if the patient is doing an active job, preferably out of doors, and he should in any case undertake an extensive and well planned exercise programme, both indoors and out.

The main points to pay attention to are breathing deeply to expand the lungs and prevent chest stiffness, bending the spine to keep it as flexible as possible, moving the legs to exercise hips and knees, and practising rotation of the neck and head so that the stiffness does not settle there. Swimming is a very good form of exercise. Movements assisted by water can be done more easily and less painfully, and most spondylitic patients get great benefit from exercising in warm swimming baths. The great emphasis, however, is on leading a generally active life which will help you to keep mobile and to keep the body as supple as possible. It is wise for someone with this condition to keep slim, as obese people are usually less active and move around less freely. Also, if a man has a stiff, aching spine, shoulders and hips the less weight he is carrying around the better.

Night is often the worst time as this is when the joints stiffen. There are

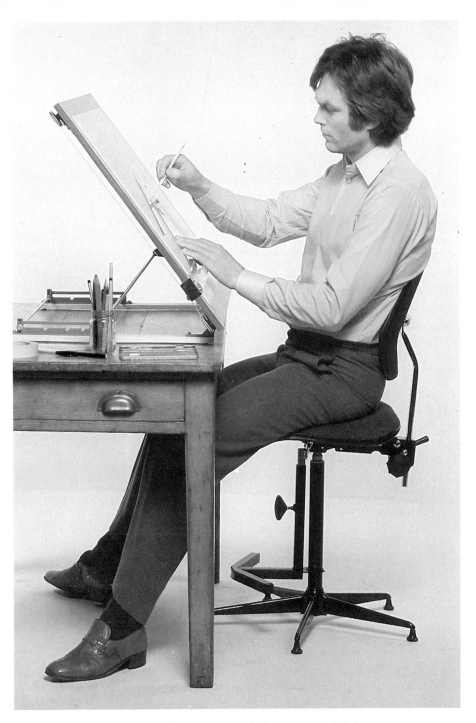

It is particularly important if you have ankylosing spondylitis to concentrate on keeping a good posture. Always sit or stand as straight as you comfortably can.

several medicines which can be given at night to diminish the pain and stiffness and to allow the sufferer to move more freely in his sleep so that he rises with less discomfort in the morning.

About 20 to 30 per cent of people with ankylosing spondylitis develop an inflammation affecting the front part of the eye known as an iritis. This responds rapidly to treatment with eye drops but it is important to note that if you get a pink, sore eye in connection with this disease you should report it promptly to your doctor.

Although in severe cases ankylosing spondylitis may affect the hips, shoulders and neck as well as the spine, it rarely afflicts the arms and legs and with all these joints intact one can still do many of the things in life. In the course of seeing many patients with ankylosing spondylitis I have always been very impressed at just how energetic they are and how much they contribute. In my experience around 80 per cent of patients who suffer from it are working full time and leading virtually normal lives, and indeed many are working harder than the rest of us. I have known several who were doing extra duties in the evening, working in boy's clubs, doing amateur theatricals, playing in concerts and so on. It is interesting to note that very few of these people become crippled. The vast majority, if allowed and encouraged to keep mobile throughout their lives, get on extremely well. Their pains are considerably helped by the various drugs available and their regular daily exercise helps them to maintain not only their mobility but their morale.

Polymyalgia rheumatica

This affects men and women over the age of fifty, the average age being sixty-five. It is entirely different from all other forms of arthritis or rheumatism and was only fully described and named in Britain in 1957. The patient notices on getting up in the morning that his or her shoulders and hips are very stiff and painful, but as the day wears on the stiffness and pain diminish. First thing in the morning it may be impossible to lift the arms above the head, whereas in the afternoon this movement may be full and almost or entirely painless. There is in most cases no swelling or pain in any other joints except the shoulder and hip girdle. To start with you will often feel ill as though you were suffering from influenza – and you may also have a fever. The disease can be very crippling and may drag on for five or six years or more. In some cases the arteries of the scalp or, more commonly, the temples are involved and become acutely inflamed and tender.

As people with polymyalgia rheumatica are usually of an age to have developed osteo-arthrosis, the diagnosis is often missed and they are considered to have just the typical changes of old age in the joints, but this is not so. A simple blood test will show in almost all cases a marked rise in sedimentation rate, and this will alert the doctor to the probability that polymyalgia rheumatica is present.

It is essentially a treatable disease, the best drug for it being one of the corticosteroids (usually prednisone or prednisolone) given in quite small doses. In most cases this will work entirely satisfactorily and both the painful shoulder and hip girdle stiffness in the morning can be rapidly controlled. Treatment should usually be kept up, at the smallest effective dosage, for several years to make sure that the condition does not relapse.

Septic arthritis

This occurs when bacteria find their way into one or more of the joints and set up an acute inflammation – rather like an abscess in the joints. Quite a large variety of bacteria can do this, one of the worst being the staphylococcus aureus, which usually causes the common boil or abscess. If you develop a boil the organism can be carried in the bloodstream from the infected site to one of your joints.

Another bacteria which does this is the gonococcus, which finds its way into the bloodstream and causes the complication of the venereal disease known as gonococal arthritis. This is an acute arthritis, usually in the knee, and the joint becomes extremely red and swollen. Happily the condition does respond rapidly to suitable medication, although some-times the pus will have to be removed by having the joint aspirated, or surgically drained. Before the 1940s gonococal arthritis was not uncommon. Then, once sulpha drugs and penicillin had become available, it disappeared almost completely, although the number of cases has recently started to rise again.

One should always beware of any hot and acutely painful joint. It can be due to all sorts of bacteria from the simple staphylococcus to rare and exotic infections, but whatever the cause the problem should be immediately reported to your doctor. It may be that you have an active infection with pus present and this could badly damage the joint if it is not rapidly diagnosed and treated. Happily, however, septic arthritis is now quite rare in many parts of the world.

Brodie's/Reiter's disease

Some inflammatory kinds of arthritis, such as the so-called colitic arthritis may be associated with chronic diarrhoea. Brodie's/Reiter's disease is a type of arthritis which follows certain types of dysentery, and it may also follow venereal disease. Brodie described four cases in London in 1818 and then, in the trenches during World War I, Hans Reiter described the case of a German cavalry officer with the disease. It is a post-infective arthritis which generally occurs two weeks or so after the original disease and in which no bacteria are actually present in the joint. It tends to affect feet and knees more than the joints of the arm but it may also affect the spine and cause a variety of ankylosing spondylitis.

Arthritis in children

Many people think of arthritis as mainly a disease of old age and do not realize that it can affect even very young children. Although it is indeed quite rare and well over 80 per cent of children with rheumatic pains are found to have something much less serious, it is nonetheless possible for a child to get arthritis.

Chronic juvenile arthritis was described by Dr George Still at the Children's Hospital, Great Ormond Street, in London some eighty years ago, and it is often known as Still's Disease. It may set in at any age, and sometimes parents first notice that one joint looks swollen or is not working properly while their child is still learning to crawl. The disease may remain restricted to one joint or it may involve several. In the large majority of cases it does burn itself out eventually, but it may take many months or even years, and throughout this time the joints must be protected by splints and exercises to make sure no permanent damage is done. It is an inflammatory arthritis and it may either come and go, getting periodically better and worse, or it may persist in a chronic form until, with luck, it eventually disappears.

A tiny percentage of children do suffer from rheumatoid arthritis and a few (mainly boys) develop ankylosing spondylitis at an early age. However, chronic juvenile arthritis is a milder disease than these and does not go on to develop into either of them.

Any children unlucky enough to develop chronic arthritis will obviously need constant help and support from their families. However they should be encouraged to remain as active as possible as this is one way they can be helped to cope with the disease on both the physical and the emotional fronts.

Bone changes

When the texture of the bone thins, this is known as osteoporosis. It is not a type of arthritis, but a condition often associated with it. It may happen after one particular area has been kept at complete rest for a long time. For instance, if you are in bed for many months or years your bones may thin from disuse. The commonest cause, however, is growing old. Elderly people's bones do become thinner, partly as a result of the aging process itself and partly because they do not get about as much as they did previously, so they miss some of the gentle daily agitation of their bones one on another which helps to keep them strong.

In women at or about the time of the menopause the spinal bones may gradually become osteoporotic and years later these patients may develop a more rounded back than the rest of womankind. Osteoporosis, however, comes to everybody as they get older and is the main reason why grandmother is perhaps a little shorter than her daughter or granddaughter. She may also become more round shouldered as she grows older, partly because of her stooping posture, partly because the cartilages in her spine lessen in thickness and also in some cases because the bones themselves contract slightly from osteoporosis. This is frequently completely painless and the woman is unaware of anything except the fact that she is becoming gradually more round shouldered and a little shorter in stature. If the bones become slightly crushed (as sometimes happens after even a trivial injury) there might be quite severe pain for several weeks or months in the bone which has sustained one of these small injuries.

Osteoporosis may occur in other bones than the spine and one reason why old ladies fall over and break the top of their femur at the hip is because the bones have become rather thinner than usual from osteoporosis. (People with osteo-arthrosis, incidentally, are less likely to develop fractured necks of their femurs as in this kind of arthritis the bones become thicker and stronger than usual – so osteo-arthrosis does perhaps have one, albeit doubtlful, benefit!)

The avoidance of osteoporosis is partly by watching your diet and partly by keeping active. You should take adequate protein and vitamins in your diet and enough calcium to preserve bone strength. The diet of an average person in the developed countries is adequate in these respects and it is usually only among certain old and immobilized patients or in some of the developing countries that many of these factors may be lacking.

The more active an elderly person is in getting around, the less likely he or she is to develop osteoporosis. Rough movements should be avoided as sudden jars and jolts may injure the bones, but gentle repetitive activity will strengthen the bones throughout your body and particularly in the spine.

3. RHEUMATISM

This rather loose and unsatisfactory term covers various different forms of inflammation, injury and disease in the connective and muscular tissue around the joints rather than in the joints themselves.

Fibrositis

In the old days fibrositis was considered to be an actual inflammation of the fibrous tissue across the shoulder areas, under and around the muscles. This was, however, probably a false assumption. Although the condition does produce considerable pain in the shoulder blades and they make peculiar noises when you move your arms, there is no direct evidence that there is any inflammatory process going on.

What does cause the pains is not fully understood, although it is likely that in many cases they are the result of arthritis in a nearby joint. Osteo-arthrosis, for instance, in the neck or between the shoulder blades may cause pains fanning out into these areas, and this is probably the most common source, but early rheumatoid arthritis may also affect the same area, as may polymyalgia rheumatica. The shoulders are also a common place for people to feel aches and pains when they are generally run down, very tired or feverish. The early start of influenza or any acute fever is often characterized by aching in the shoulder girdle.

Fibrositis is a great nuisance, but not a serious disease. It does not cause any changes in the blood and it is not dangerous. Treatment usually takes the form of exercises, warmth and rubs with liniments and ointments. These help relieve the pain even if they do not actually remove it, and it will eventually cease of its own accord.

Tennis or golfer's elbow

This usually begins as a result of a small tear or an area of degeneration in the muscles at the elbow. It can be very painful and take many months to heal, but heal it does eventually. Injections of cortisone are often given to hurry the process along but they do not always help. The disease is a nuisance as it restricts the use of your arm and interferes with many other

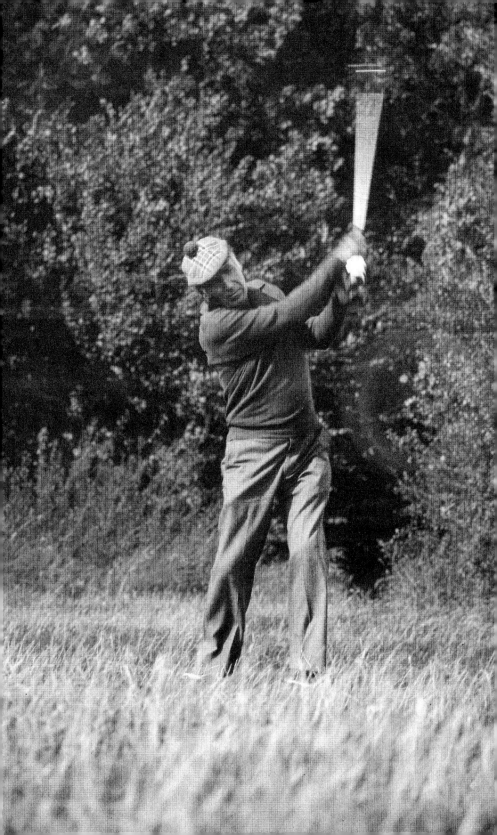

activities besides sport. It is important, if you suffer from it, to avoid forceful movements and to stop playing tennis or golf as otherwise the pain very often persists or returns. It is best, in other words, to play for time rather than for a cup or gold medal, and to use the joint less than usual.

The painful shoulder

This can be due to a number of disorders. It can follow a strain or injury or may just appear out of the blue for no apparent reason. All sorts of arthritis can also of course involve the shoulder, including rheumatoid arthritis which affects the shoulder joint itself, and osteo-arthrosis which tends to affect the joint between the collar bone and the shoulder blade.

The pain usually arises not in the joints themselves but in the soft tissue or tendons around them, where small areas of injury or degeneration occur. X-rays may later show calcium salts deposited there. Raising your arm to beyond a right angle is very often impossible because it is too agonising and movement in all directions is restricted or painful.

Like the tennis elbow, a painful shoulder can take a long time (perhaps one or two years) to get better spontaneously, but in the end it almost invariably does. An injection of cortisone often helps it to heal more quickly but in some cases it does not work and if the injection is into the tendon itself it may sometimes injure or even rupture it. On the whole it is better to treat the shoulder gently and to rest the arm rather than to exercise it vigorously, as being too energetic with such a joint can damage it and make it stiffer and more painful than before. The best answer may be to wear a sling to look Admiral Nelson on his flag ship, *Victory*, or to rest your shoulder by tucking your arm under your coat over your stomach, like Napoleon at the battle of Waterloo.

One hears a lot about 'frozen shoulders'. Strictly speaking this term should be used for a shoulder that is fused or stuck and is so stiff that it is physically impossible to move it fully or at all. However people often use the word to mean simply that they cannot move their shoulder because it is too painful, although as soon as the pain wears off movement returns.

What you should do

1. If you have an injury or pain in your shoulder it is as well to see your doctor and make sure that you have not got arthritis or a fracture or, if you are over sixty, polymyalgia rheumatica (see page 40). It is much more likely to be just a painful or 'frozen' shoulder but it is a good idea to have it checked.

2. Be patient. Rome wasn't built in a day, and the painful shoulder can take a long time to recover – but in the end it will.

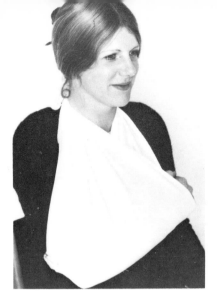

A simple sling like this can bring relief to a painful shoulder.

3. Rest your shoulder as much as possible and only use your arm within the range where it does not feel painful. It is better to use some kind of sling or support than to leave the arm dangling down. Avoid carrying heavy weights with the affected arm.

4. Heat treatments, such as a hot water bottle in a thick cover or an electric pad, can help relieve the pain. A few patients prefer a cold pack, but most seem to find that heat works better.

5. Backward movement of the arm is usually very painful so when dressing it is a good idea to get someone to help you put on things such as coats. If you put your arm into the sleeve first, the helper can slide the coat on for you. Aprons and bras are best fastened in front and then swung round to the back.

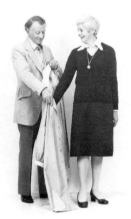
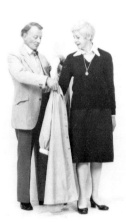
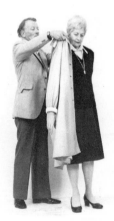

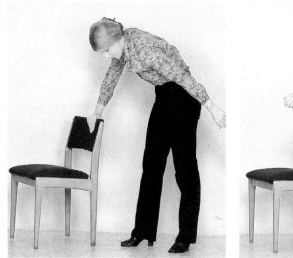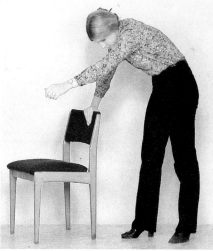

A gentle exercise for the painful shoulder (see below).

6. Although any vigorous exercise will make the problem worse, it can be helpful to take your shoulder *gently* through as full a range of movement as you can two or three times a day. Swing your arm very gently forwards, backwards and sideways, but not pushing past the point of acute pain. This may be easier and less painful to do after a hot bath or shower. Just move the arm as far as you can and try to maintain, or very gradually extend, your range as time goes by. As the pains improve exercises can be done more frequently and the movements increased. If the pain and stiffness return, ease off again. One good method is to use gravity assisted exercises. Lean down, resting your good arm on a table or the back of a chair. Then let your other arm hang free until it begins to feel heavy. Swing it gently to and fro from the shoulder, keeping your elbow straight. But be patient. Don't force the pace, as over-vigorous manipulations will often actually set you back.

7. It is important to adjust your pillow at night so that your head and neck are in a comfortable position and you avoid putting too much pressure on the painful shoulder. You may also find it helpful to rest the arm on a pillow and a little experimenting will probably establish what position is least painful. Sedatives and pain killers prescribed by your doctor may be necessary at night and, if pains are severe, during the day.

Back ache

This is one of mankind's most troublesome complaints. The spine is a crazy structure with twenty-four vertebrae all balanced on top of each

48

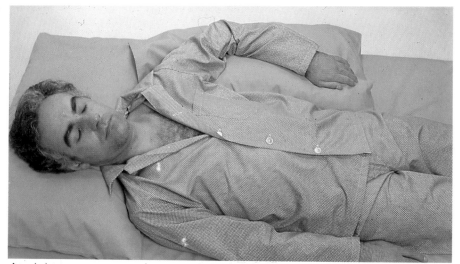

At night you can sometimes ease a painful shoulder by resting your arm over an extra pillow.

other, and a joint between each one. On top of the column is the heavy weight of the skull. All in all it is not surprising that pain, injuries or diseases of the spinal column are amongst the most widespread of human ailments. Most often the problems arise either in the neck (cervical spine) or the lower back (lumbar spine).

Neck pains

These may be due to simple injuries or twists, in which case they get better fairly rapidly. The so called 'wry neck', for example, when you have to hold your head tilted over towards the shoulder usually settles down

Butterfly pillow: To help an aching neck try tying a bandage round your pillow to make this comfortable butterfly shape.

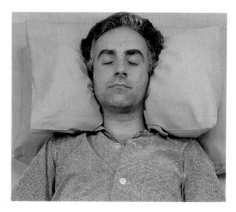
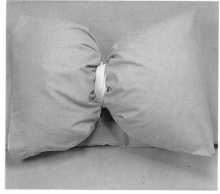

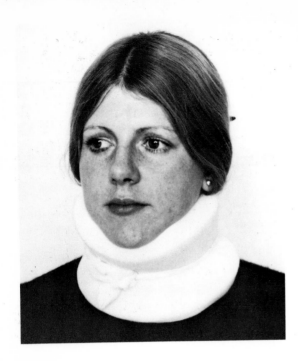

Left Soft collars can be an excellent support for a painful neck.

Right **Neck exercises:** Moving your head gently left, right and up and down several times can help restore movement to a stiff neck.

within a few days. However, when degenerative changes or osteo-arthrosis occur in the joints and in the discs between the vertebrae of the neck, the pain may be worse and last longer. As you get older the joints in your neck become gradually stiffer and pains may fan out from them into the back of your head and shoulders.

If the pain is very severe you will have to rest at home flat on a bed with only a light support for your head. A bandage tied round the pillow allowing the neck to rest in the 'V' is often comfortable and several small pillows packed in and around the neck help to immobilize it. As soon as the acute pain has settled you can get up and start moving around, but you may be grateful at this stage for the support of either a firm or a soft felt collar. Generally the soft collars are more popular. But a word of caution is in order here. You should not go on wearing a collar too long as this may weaken the muscles and make your condition worse.

Quite often simple neck traction or pulling on the head is very helpful, but this is a manoeuvre that has to be done by a physiotherapist or a doctor who is expert in the field – amateur traction is not to be encouraged. There are also simple forms of heat treatment and exercises which can be done at home, but if more than this is required you should consult your doctor. Gentle neck exercises turning your head each way to look first to the left and then to the right as far as you can, or leaning your head sideways onto each shoulder in turn, can help the neck recover.

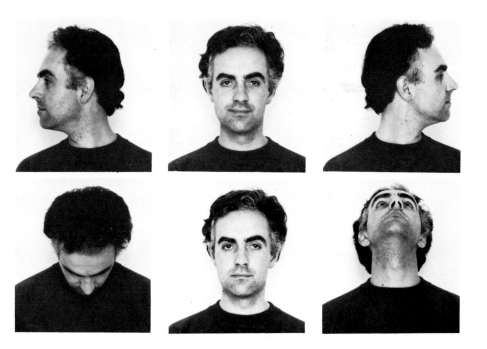

Lumbar back ache

This kind of low back pain is extremely common. It is sometimes due to an injury or sprain and sometimes occurs because one of the small discs has protruded between the vertebrae and is pressing on a nerve root, ligament or some other sensitive area nearby. When the pain radiates down one leg it may be because the disc has pressed on a nerve root.

The best initial treatment, if possible, is to rest on a firm mattress, if necessary with a board beneath it to make the bed really stable, and with one supporting pillow. Sometimes two mattresses are needed to take some of the hardness out of the board beneath. The more one wrestles on with severe back ache by insisting on returning to work and 'keeping going', the longer it tends to last and the worse it gets. Most back aches respond to rest and when the acute symptoms settle down you can gradually start to move about again and then later return to your normal duties. Unfortunately, many people with back ache leap out of bed whenever the telephone goes or the front door bell rings and do not give their poor spines a chance to recover.

Manipulation may sometimes have dramatic effects, but as several sessions are often necessary it may well be that in many cases it is time rather than the manipulation that has helped the back most. Almost all lumbar backaches get better given time, especially if enough rest and pain-killing medicines are given in the early stages. Traction, that is pulling on the legs with the help of a form of harness, can also be helpful but is best done in hospital. Exercises to strengthen the stomach muscles can help the lower back considerably.

Very few low back aches need surgery. Well over 90 per cent recover as a result of simple home measures and a period of absolute rest, although the recovery may take a few weeks or sometimes much longer.

How to prevent it

Once a back ache, you might say, always a potential back ache. If your back has given trouble perhaps even ten or twenty years ago, you should always be on the alert and take special care of it as the problem could be triggered off again at any time by a rough or unnatural movement. Very often lifting weights, or even something small and light such as a pencil, with the spine bent will cause the pain to return. A sudden jolt or twisting movement such as getting out of a car can also precipitate it.

Ordinary daily life puts a great strain on our backs, particularly if we find ourselves having to stand in one position for a long time. Domestic chores such as washing up, cooking, ironing, making beds or digging in the garden can all bring on or aggravate back pain, and should be done in the way that puts the least possible strain on the spine. When making beds, for example, it is better to kneel on the floor than to stoop down over the bed. Likewise, if you have to pick up something heavy you should always do so with your spine straight, so that your legs, hips and knees do the bending rather than your back.

There is another book in this series called *The Back – Relief from Pain* by Dr Alan Stoddard which discusses the problem of back ache in detail.

Muscles

Many aches and pains appear to arise in the muscles. Muscles may indeed be painful when they are torn or injured or in tight spasm, but in most cases the pains are referred to the muscles from bones, joints and ligaments elsewhere. For instance, pains in the thigh muscles which feel as if they are arising from the knee are often in fact caused by arthritis in the hip. Likewise, muscular pains around the hip are often the result of degenerative changes in the base of the spine. The fact that the site of the pain appears to be in the muscles does not mean that it necessarily arises from there. There is an inflammatory disease of muscles called myositis or polymyositis, but this condition is relatively rare. Most aches and pains are due to problems not in the muscles themselves but in nearby joints.

When a joint is diseased and cannot function normally and is painful, stiff and perhaps swollen, the muscles serving it tend to waste and become

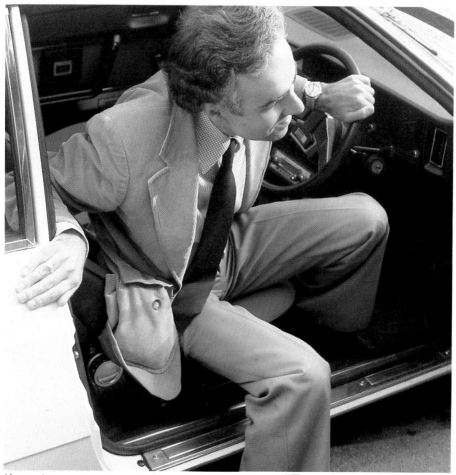

If you have a tendency to back pain always take special care over awkward, twisting movements such as getting out of a car.

Wrong:

Right: Always pick up heavy weights with your spine as upright as possible.

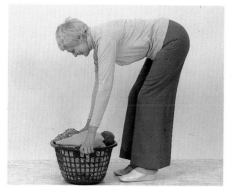

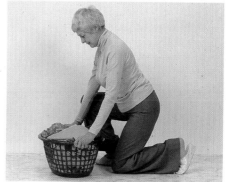

thinner and weaker. One sees this best in the case of an arthritic knee, where the muscles in the thigh become weaker, smaller and less strong. In a way this is a function of nature. The joint should not be over-used when it is diseased and the muscles weaken, but as soon as the joint returns to normal the muscles come gradually back to their usual strength and size. When muscles serving an arthritic joint waste a little it is therefore not entirely a bad thing as it does diminish the tendency for the patient to over-use the affected joint.

Tendons

These are the thin strong ends of the muscles where they are inserted into the bones, usually not far distant from the joints. They contain nerve endings and are therefore much more sensitive than the muscles themselves. Normally they move smoothly and effortlessly in their own small, surrounding sheaths. You can feel them for example at the base of your thumb when you move it back and forth, or at the wrist when you make piano playing movements with your fingers. They are more readily strained and sprained than the muscle bodies themselves.

The biggest one in the body can be felt just above the ankle at the back of the lower part of the calf. This is the so-called Achilles tendon. In spite of the fact that it is the largest and strongest tendon in the body, it does quite often get ruptured, usually when playing tennis or squash. A sudden violent jerk will tear the ligament right across, and it can sometimes also rupture after an injection has been made directly into it.

Other tendons may also snap across, for instance those in your hand, which run down the back and front of the fingers. If you rupture a tendon in your palm the end results, even with satisfactory and early operation, are not always perfect and the fingers may subsequently be rather stiff and difficult to move. But a rupture of the extensor tendon down the back of the fingers can usually be operated on with excellent results. At the shoulder there are a number of tendons running down into the arm and these again can easily get injured, and the so-called painful or frozen shoulder may result (see page 46). A ruptured tendon can be operated on but the only thing you can do with a strained tendon is to rest it until it heals of its own accord.

Nerves

Nerves run from the spinal cord to every part of the body, but some structures are more richly supplied with nerves and nerve endings than others. The cartilages, for instance, are not particularly sensitive but the ligaments and the capsules of the joints are extremely so and no part of the body is completely insensitive. A nerve may become inflamed or compressed, and this disease is called a neuritis or neuropathy. The best example is sciatica. The sciatic nerve, which runs down the thigh from the back of the buttock and the lower part of the spine, is the largest nerve in the body. If it is pressed on by, for example, a damaged disc in the spine, you get an extremely unpleasant pain running down the back and buttock into one leg. Often the reflexes of the leg are then affected and you may get areas of numbness in the outer lower part of the shin just above the ankle.

Neuritis can be due to a large number of conditions. Diabetics, for instance, tend to get numb feet due to degenerative changes in the nerves of the area. The same thing occasionally happens to people with rheumatoid arthritis and, not so rarely, to people who drink far too much alcohol over long periods. However, many conditions described as neuritis are not really so, but are merely a pain referred from some other part of the body. Many cases of so-called sciatica, for instance, are really pains due to arthritis, or some other disease or injury, in the lower part of the spine.

One most unpleasant form of neuritis, where there is actual inflammation of a nerve, is shingles, an infection which usually affects a nerve in one area on just one side of the body. At first there is a very acute pain, sharp burning or stinging, usually in the chest or abdomen, radiating round in a narrow band. This is followed a day or two later by the typical rash or blisters of shingles. It is a virus infection and usually passes off rapidly. However, in the case of elderly people, the nerve often remains scarred and painful and the poor patient suffers for many months, or even in a few cases for years, from persistent pain in the area of the nerve. It is called Herpes Zoster after two Greek words meaning 'to creep' and 'girdle', as it is like a snake biting its way round one side of the body. Even more unpleasant is when it affects the head and scalp on one side and also, very rarely, the front of the eye. However it never crosses the midline and is always limited to just one side of the body.

Pain killers will probably be necessary in the acute stages of the disease. It can be very uncomfortable to have anything in contact with the sensitive area and so it helps to have loose bedclothes and clothing which will not rub or stick to the skin.

Bursae

Bursa is Latin for purse, or small bag. We have seventy-eight such bursae each side of the body, some of them very small and some as large as 3 inches (75 mm) across. They are usually invisible and you are not aware of them unless they become inflamed or distended with fluid in which case

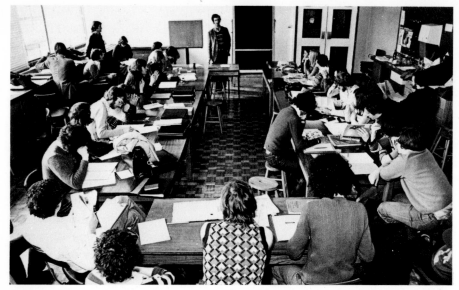

Student's elbow: Bursitis in the elbows can begin as a result of leaning them too long on hard surfaces – so students are particularly at risk!

they show as swelling in different parts of the body, although they are not usually very painful.

The purpose of a bursa is to act as a shock absorber or cushion between different bones and tendons. There are, for instance, small ones between the bones at the base of the toes, so that each bone can move easily against the next one when you walk.

Bursitis merely means inflammation of one or other of the bursae in the body. The bursa in front of the knee cap may become swollen and inflamed from too much kneeling (Housemaid's, Nun's or Priest's knee). One over the point of the elbow may do so as a result of repeated pressing on a hard surface, for example student's elbow (after leaning on a desk) and boozer's elbow (after leaning on a bar). One form of bursitis which was not uncommon in the old days was the so-called 'Weaver's Bottom', which affected the pelvic bones after someone had spent a long time sitting on hard surfaces while weaving chair seats.

In an inflammatory arthritis, such as rheumatoid arthritis, the bursae may become inflamed as part of the disease process and contribute to the swelling around the joints, particularly in knee, shoulder and elbow. However, bursitis is rarely a major trouble in itself and although it can occasionally cause pain, discomfort and considerable swelling, it will usually settle without treatment. The bursae can be injected with cortisone or removed by surgery if they become a serious nuisance, but this is rarely necessary.

4. WHAT CAUSES OR AFFECTS ARTHRITIS?

Many factors can play a part in the development of arthritis, including heredity, hormones (as, for example, in the kinds of arthritis which appear after the menopause), and infections of one sort and another. One major cause is injury. Repeated minor injuries, such as damage caused to the big toe by wearing badly fitting shoes or to the hands by rough usage, can add up over the years in some cases to cause degenerative changes in the joints. There are doubtless many other factors, but as yet the causes of most sorts of arthritis are still not fully understood. Further studies and research will, we hope, give us some more of the answers before very long.

In most cases there is little you can do in order to prevent the onset of arthritis. There is, for instance, no sure way of stopping degenerative changes from taking place in the body or of preventing the development of a disease such as rheumatoid arthritis. As we grow older our cartilages and other tissues become less elastic and the longer we live the more likely we are to suffer repeated injuries to them. It is too much to hope for an elixir of youth. Permanent youth will never be with us and this is probably just as well. However, there are some ways in which, by paying attention to our general health and lifestyle, we can at least improve our ability to withstand the onslaught of arthritis or of the mechanical insults or cross-infections which could trigger it off.

Many myths have arisen about what influences the onset and development of arthritis and this chapter will examine some of the numerous factors which have been associated with it and try to distinguish the old wives' tales from those which have an element of truth.

The weather

Almost any sufferer from arthritis feels certain that it is affected by cold and damp. There is in fact no good evidence that weather conditions can actually cause any form of arthritis and the disease is as common in the Sahara or in Florida as it is in more arctic regions. Having said this, it is nonetheless true that bad weather can certainly make most pains and aches feel worse. A cold grey day makes the spirits grey also, and any symptom will seem more noticeable when you are feeling depressed.

Changes in barometric pressure, either up or down, do undoubtedly aggravate the pains in arthritis, even though they may not affect the underlying disease. I knew of a man who had had his arm amputated but claimed to be able to tell from the feeling in the stump of his arm whenever the weather was changing. Cold draughts playing on a muscle may set up muscle pains and spasm. For example, motorists travelling with an open car window and with a cold draught blowing on the side of their necks often experience discomfort and stiffness as a result. In hot countries over-exposure to air conditioning or sitting in cold draughts may also set up muscle pains.

Cold air contracts the blood vessels by acting, indirectly, on the muscles in their walls. (The so-called 'goose flesh' you get when cold is due to the small muscles in the skin contracting.) Warmth relaxes both muscles and mind and so, even though it does not have any effect on the arthritic condition itself, it can soothe away some of the pain.

A few people prefer cool weather to hot and humid days, but they are the exceptions. Most commonly it is the wet, penetrating cold air that seems to have the worst effect. In general someone with arthritis will gain great benefit from a sunny summer holiday. Relaxing in warm, pleasant surroundings not only makes you feel generally much better but very often does also help the arthritic symptoms to subside.

Chilly draughts, as for example when you are driving with an open window, can sometimes give you aches and pains, but cold weather cannot cause arthritis.

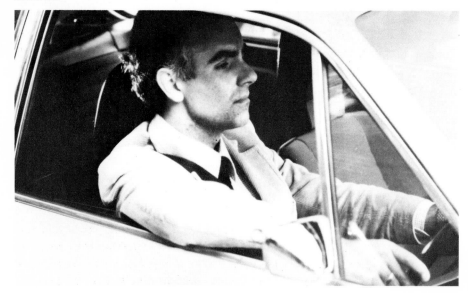

Heredity

Children tend to take after their parents or grandparents in many ways so it is not surprising if some forms of arthritis appear to run in families. It is, for instance, not uncommon to find a son developing gout when he reaches middle age if his father did so at about the same age. Another example is ankylosing spondylitis, where people of a certain tissue type appear predisposed to the disease. If a child happens to have the particular tissue antigen from birth he is that much more likely to develop the condition. However even among people who have this tissue type it is only the minority who do in fact develop ankylosing spondylitis. Another condition which appears to be hereditary is generalized osteo-arthrosis, which is seen most commonly in post-menopausal women and does occur more often in some families than others.

It seems as though some people have better cartilages than others, and those with first class cartilages, so to speak, are less likely to suffer from osteo-arthrosis. This characteristic may be something which runs in families, but there are many common types of osteo-arthrosis which do not seem to have any hereditary element. Rheumatoid arthritis is likewise not an inherited disease and few families have more than one member who suffers from it.

Young couples about to marry may, if one of them is affected by some form of arthritis, wonder what the likelihood is that their children will have the same disease. This will depend not only on the type of arthritis in question, but also on how many of their forebears have suffered from it. In the case of gout 20 per cent of people with an immediate relative who has the disease will go on to develop it. For ankylosing spondylitis this figure is only 10 per cent. If the same kind of arthritis is present in both families then the risk may be further increased. However, there is still only an off chance that any children will have the disease. It is not like haemophilia where any male children born of haemophilic stock are very likely indeed to inherit it. With most kinds of arthritis the risk that a child will develop it may be greater than average if there is a family history of the disease, but it remains a small risk and certainly should not be great enough to deter anyone from having children.

Diet

Arthritis has only very rarely been directly associated with dietetic factors. There is a disorder called Kashin-Beck or Urov disease which appeared in Russia and Northern China some years ago and was apparently associated with fungal infection of cereal grain, but this is rapidly disappearing and is

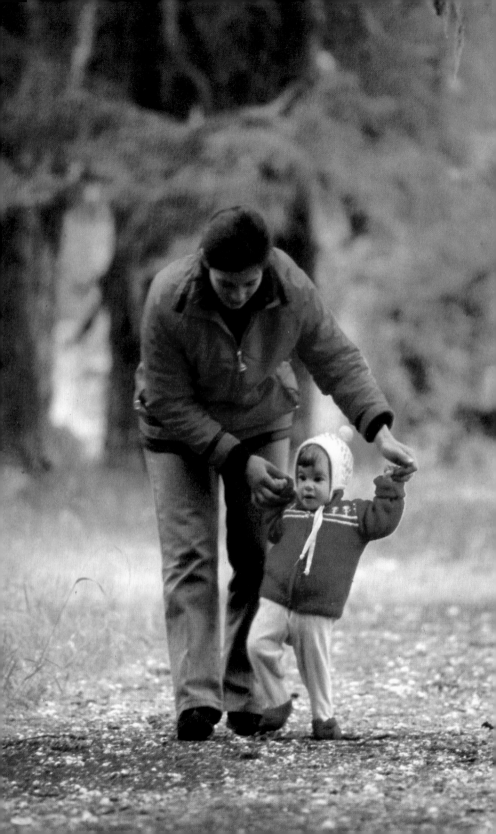

now very rare. Other forms of arthritis are not directly caused or influenced by food and there is no one diet that is suitable for all of them.

However there is no doubt that obesity is very bad for an arthritic patient, and getting the right balance of calories, neither too much nor too little, is essential. Fat people tend to take less exercise, move their joints less and become generally less healthy. Besides this a person with arthritis may find the pain is worse and he will be less mobile if he has an excessive amount of weight bearing down on his joints.

Fats, sugars, starches, potatoes, pastries, bread, rice and any fried foods are the first things you should cut down on if you tend to gain weight excessively. Most adults do not need more than one good meal or a few smaller ones each day with plenty of fresh fruit and vegetables, but this does depend on their occupation. Lumberjacks, for instance, need far more calories than office workers, and people's diets should be gauged accordingly. High animal fats are rather out of fashion today and many people fear that their blood fat levels are too high. As animal fats do in any case contain many calories it is wise to cut down on them if you want to slim.

Alcohol contains a large number of calories and may cause obesity if taken to excess. An occasional drink does no great harm, but patients with rheumatoid arthritis often find that taking more than a small amount of alcohol makes them feel worse.

Male and female hormones

Many forms of arthritis affect one sex more than the other. Certain types of osteo-arthrosis are more common in men, others in women. The post-menopausal generalized osteo-arthrosis, for instance, is naturally more common in women and the type of osteo-arthrosis which results from rough, hard use of the joints and particularly affects manual workers is more common in men. Gout is essentially a male disease and it seems as though the female hormones prevent its development, since if women do get gout it is usually after the menopause when their hormone balance has changed. The uric acid in the blood, which is the cause of gout, only rises to abnormally high levels in men when they reach puberty and, in those few women who later develop gout, after the menopause. Rheumatoid arthritis on the other hand is three times more common in women than it is in men. Ankylosing spondylitis mainly affects males, particularly in its fully developed form, and if women do get it it is usually in a milder version.

It seems that the male and female hormones do tend to prevent certain forms of arthritis in one or other sex. The lessening of female hormone levels at the menopause tends in women to lead to a general reduction in the strength and density of the bones (see *Bone changes*, page 42). In men this occurs with old age and in certain rare conditions where male hormone levels are diminished. (In some instances male hormones are used therapeutically to strengthen bones.) However exactly why there should be a connection between some kind of arthritis and male and female hormones is something which is not yet fully understood.

Lack of exercise

Joints that are never moved tend to become stiff and therefore more likely to develop disorders. I am constantly amazed, when doing routine examinations on middle aged men, by how restricted they are in their movements, particularly of the spine and hips. Many men of only fifty or fifty-five years of age have lost up to 25 per cent of their normal range of movement. They can still flex their hip to a right angle since they exercise that action when sitting down every day, but in other ways the hip is gradually stiffening and the movements diminishing from disuse.

Exercise every day, therefore, is important, preferably out of doors where the stimulus of fresh air is good for both soul and body. Walking in fresh air every day, moving all your muscles, is a form of exercise taken by far too few people, although the recent popularity of jogging around

If your job means you have to sit at a desk for much of the day regular exercise is especially important to keep your hips and other joints from getting stiff.

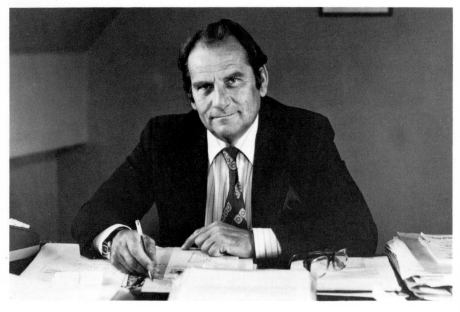

parks and back streets is a step or, more literally, many steps in the right direction.

Along with exercise go exercises, and every joint should be moved through its full range of movement several times each day in order to keep the body supple and in its best working order. Detailed suggestions on exercising are given in the next chapter on pages 70 to 76.

Arthritis and the bowels

Some years ago everybody felt quite sure that constipation caused all sorts of unpleasant diseases, and operations were done to remove large portions of the gut as it was believed that various poisons lurked there that would be best removed. Constipation, in fact, often has no side-effects whatsoever and can be easily avoided by eating a high-fibre diet. Some patients are unpleasantly aware of their colons if their bowels do not move regularly but there is no evidence that constipation causes, or even aggravates, any of the different kinds of arthritis.

On the other hand patients with some forms of chronic diarrhoea (for instance, those with ulcerative colitis) can sometimes be especially prone to develop pain and swelling in some of the joints although why is not certain. There is evidence that infections of the gut, particularly in people with certain tissue types, can bring on spinal arthritis, but this only applies to a small subgroup of sufferers. In most cases the bowels have little to do with arthritis of any sort and, while constipation and diarrhoea may cause the arthritic patient some additional discomforts, they are unlikely in most cases to make the arthritis itself any worse.

Skin conditions

There are a few forms of arthritis which are associated with specific skin conditions. The most common example is psoriatic arthritis, which affects about 5 to 10 per cent of patients who have the chronic skin disease known as psoriasis. As a rule the arthritis will only appear many years after the psoriasis and will affect the joints in the arms and legs, although it can also occasionally cause stiffness in the spine. Psoriasis seems to run in families and about a third of the people who suffer from it have a parent or other relative with the disease. Why these people should be vulnerable to this particular type of arthritis is not known. The arthritis and the skin condition do not develop simultaneously, and sometimes the psoriasis may improve as the arthritis worsens or vice versa.

In addition there are some kinds of arthritis which may have skin conditions as part of their symptoms. Children with Still's disease (see page

42) may develop certain rashes, as may children with rheumatic fever. Septic arthritis, where the bacterial invasion of the joint is often part of a generalized infection going right through the body and the bloodstream, may also be accompanied by septic spots and abscesses on the skin.

Infections

Some forms of arthritis are caused by acute infections and, while it is not easy to take active steps to avoid catching these, there is no doubt that the quick control of an infection in its early stages may make all the difference between a prolonged low grade illness and a quick recovery. It is perhaps very virtuous and stoical to struggle on and continue to work when you feel like dropping, but what you are often in fact doing is spreading the infection to other people and doing yourself no good at the same time. It is sometimes wiser to have a day or two off and take medicine to conquer the problem as fast as possible. Unfortunately most such cross-infections are due to viruses and there is often no quick cure, but suitable antibiotics may control the secondary infections which otherwise prolong your illness after the acute symptoms have ended.

Rheumatic fever among children always followed a certain infection and there is no doubt that eradicating particular bacteria that has been a factor in the prevention of this disease which is now much less often seen in the developed countries. Septic arthritis, another rare disease, is also prevented by treating infections early and efficiently.

Rheumatoid and many other kinds of inflammatory arthritis may be made worse by cross-infections which often seem to 'stir up' the arthritic condition. Anybody with chronic arthritis of any sort has plenty to cope with as it is without the added burden of an infection, and so the prevention or early cure of such ailments becomes doubly important.

Repeated small injuries

Osteo-arthrosis can follow not only from a large injury such as a strain or a broken bone, but also from repeated, unnecessary small injuries accumulated day by day. A predisposition to osteo-arthrosis may depend on something as hard to pin down as the expertness or otherwise with which you carry out the ordinary daily routines of your life. The way you make a bed, the way you sit and work at a table or desk, or many other similar activities in office or home or factory can, with a little extra care, be done so as to cause the minimum stress to the muscles and joints involved, and even these small precautions could perhaps help your joints to stay healthier for longer.

Growing pains

In the old days people used to be very worried about these, but a study done in London before World War Two showed that only a very small percentage of children who had so-called growing pains developed any form of arthritis. Usually the aches and pains around the knees, hips, back and elsewhere, were just part of growing up, although in some cases other factors were present such as badly fitting shoes, poor nutrition, bad posture, general ill health or a hearty dislike of going to school. Only in under 5 per cent was any true rheumatism or arthritis detected. (Juvenile arthritis is discussed on page 42.)

Nevertheless the same principles on avoiding arthritis apply to children as to their parents. Bad posture, badly designed shoes or tight socks all tend to deform the joints, even though body tissues are more elastic and adaptable in children than they are in adults.

Rheumatic fever was a common disease in the last century, but it began to diminish after World War One and is now rare in the developed countries. It was a dangerous disease for children, not because of the arthritis (which usually disappeared in a few weeks) but because it damaged the heart. The serious importance of flitting pains to an Edwardian or

Most children get growing pains at some time or other but these are hardly ever a sign that anything is wrong.

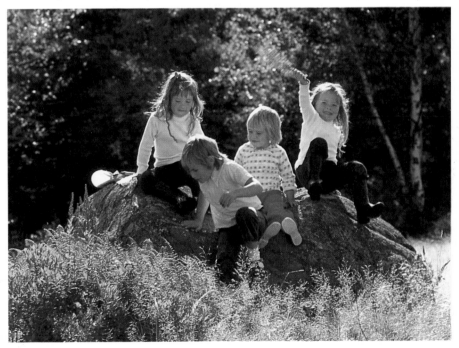

Victorian mother was the possibility that her child might be developing rheumatic fever. Today, with our improved living conditions and the advent of effective new drugs, this is a very small risk indeed.

Joint noises and 'double joints'

Many people are concerned about noises in the joints. Some children make noises with their fingers and wrists as a kind of party trick. Some are even 'double jointed' and enjoy moving their hands or feet into abnormal positions. They should be encouraged not to do so as any repeated strain is bad for the joints, and certainly deliberately producing noises from them does neither performer nor audience any good!

As you get older you can often hear different joints moving – for example your knees may creak when you go downstairs, or your neck when you turn your head sideways and so on, but these noises matter very little. Almost everybody over the age of fifty can sometimes hear noises when they move and this does not mean that their joints are diseased in any way. It is not noises that matter, but only pain or restricted movement. Some people are aware of a constant rheumatic calypso band as they move around, but although this may be quite dramatic if the record is played for visitors, it has very little relevance to general health.

5. TREATMENTS

Can arthritis be cured?

Some types of arthritis, such as rheumatic fever and septic arthritis, can be prevented by improving social conditions and eradicating the infection which causes them, and can be cured with readily accessible drugs. Other sorts, such as gout and polymyalgia rheumatica, can be effectively controlled by medical treatment. Inflammatory kinds of arthritis of unknown cause, such as rheumatoid, cannot as yet be cured and the best that can be done is to lessen the pain, to prevent the muscles and joints from contracting or becoming deformed, and to maintain as much as possible of the patient's function and morale. In these diseases a natural remission or cure can often occur, and even in a chronic condition such as osteo-arthrosis the disorder settles down and the pains may lessen or go away, sometimes for a very long time. Painful back aches and soft tissue rheumatisms may also be agonising for a time and then disappear completely and for ever.

Many kinds of rheumatism do settle down largely or completely in time and it is only the nasty few that go relentlessly on. This is the reason why so many false cures are claimed, as whatever treatment is being taken at the time the arthritis settles down often gets the credit, whether it be a new pill or a new diet or a new nature cure, and whether or not it has actually had any beneficial effect.

There are certain specific treatments for particular kinds of arthritis which are dealt with in chapters two and three, but there are also a number of general points that can be made on coping with arthritis and relieving arthritic pain, and these are discussed below.

Mental attitude

This is one of the most important aspects of tackling and conquering arthritis. It is very bad luck if you develop the disorder but you cannot blame it on anyone or anything and it quite definitely makes things very much worse if you continue to feel resentful and bewail your ill fortune. The best patients are those who accept their condition and get on with living their lives in a modified way which will not aggravate or worsen the pain and stiffness.

Optimism and faith are perhaps the arthritic's greatest secret weapon. Giving way and getting depressed or throwing in the sponge will lose you the fight, but a good programme of therapy and a positive attitude towards your disability are the best ways of rising above it. I must say, I am constantly amazed at the large numbers of uncomplaining rheumatic and arthritic saints there are in the world, compared with the small minority of grumblers and complainers. It is often the worst affected who make the fewest complaints and, because they have a positive attitude towards their disability, do best in the end.

Learning to live with pain

The pain threshold, or in other words the point at which an unpleasant stimulus becomes actual pain, is something which varies widely from one individual to another. Some people are natural stoics. They have high pain thresholds and a stimulus has to be very marked before they will consider it painful. They will shrug off even a heart attack as mere indigestion and go on gardening or ploughing the fields. On the other hand, people with low thresholds feel pains at levels that ordinary people would not. They experience frequent discomforts throughout the day and tend to consume a large number of pain-killing tablets. This pain threshold is in part a matter of personality and in part a result of upbringing. Some children are taught to be stoics and not complain unless their aches and pains are very persistent or severe. Others, with mothers who are perhaps too sympathetic, rush immediately to the aspirin bottle as soon as they feel the slightest twinge. Most people, happily, are between these two extremes.

There is no doubt that all of us suffer small unpleasant sensations on and off throughout the day, particularly as we get older. As you sit quietly in your chair, ask yourself what unpleasant things you can feel going on in your body. It is often amazing how many you notice if you think about it, but most of us suppress them automatically at source. If the mind is occupied with other things, what we might call silly pains are not recognized as such and can be ignored. This kind of minor pain control is a good semi-conscious self-discipline and helps us cope with our daily discomforts.

At a certain point of course the recognition of pain can serve a useful purpose by alerting us to the fact that something is wrong which we should correct. For instance, after you have been sitting in a certain position for long enough to feel uncomfortable you move so as to take the strain from the affected ligaments. Beyond this point, however, and particularly with a chronic pain such as arthritis, the degree of discomfort ceases to give you any useful guidance as to what to do about it. In this case developing a stoical philosophy and finding ways to conquer or forget about the pain is of far greater value to you than constantly resorting to the medicine bottle.

One of the best ways of forgetting about minor pains is to occupy your mind by thinking about things outside your own body. People with no distractions feel far more pain than those who are busy and interested in achieving outside goals. This is one reason why pains can seem worse at night, once everything is dark and your mind may have nothing else to think about except your sufferings.

Analgesics and anti-rheumatic drugs are extremely helpful not only in relieving pain but also in reducing inflammation in the tissues. In most cases these drugs are absolutely necessary and there is no special virtue in enduring pain for the sake of it. But the drugs should nonetheless be taken in the smallest amount needed to control the pain and make it possible for you to get through the day's activities. Remember that any medicine, whatever its virtues, also has the power to do you harm. The essential thing is to follow your doctor's instructions exactly, as he will control the dose to suit your needs. Always remember that if you start to take the drugs erratically or change the dose without his advice this will not help you and could even be dangerous.

Exercise

The amount of exercise you should do will vary according to which kind of arthritis you have got and the severity of your symptoms. Getting the right balance between exercise and rest is important and some guidance on this in relation to specific forms of arthritis is given in chapters two and three. Any very acute arthritis must be rested as the joints will be too swollen and painful for you to do anything else, but as soon as the acute pain lessens gentle exercise should be started as all joints will benefit from being kept as supple and mobile as possible.

Outdoor exercise is particularly good, and walking on soft surfaces such as grass is preferable to hard roads or rough, uneven surfaces – although if you live in a city you may have no choice in this matter. When taking such outdoor exercise, you should spread your wings gradually and increase your range week by week – but remember you have to fly home! The return journey may be painful if you have been too adventurous. Particularly in the case of an inflammatory condition such as rheumatoid arthritis where the weight-bearing joints are swollen and painful, it is best to be less ambitious and err on the side of going a shorter distance than you think you can manage.

Daily exercises or 'operation de-freeze'

Besides the great benefits of leading a generally active and healthy life, it is also valuable for an arthritic patient to do daily exercises aimed at keeping specific joints from becoming stiff and restricted. These exercises should be done morning and evening, and ideally when you are warm and glowing from a hot shower or bath. Certain leg and arm movements can actually be performed while you are in the bath. Any exercise programme you follow should be done under the guidance of your physiotherapist who will make sure it is suitable for your individual case.

You should aim gradually to extend your exercises so that each day you get a little more movement in the affected part, but do not push forward too hard or too enthusiastically as this may result in a relapse. A good general rule is that, whatever form of exercise or physiotherapy you are doing, if your joints ache for a few minutes afterwards then this does not matter, but if the increased pain and stiffness last for more than an hour you should reduce the amount of exercise next time.

Muscles always waste to some extent when a joint is inflamed. If the knee, for instance, has active rheumatoid arthritis, the muscles above it tend to become weaker and smaller than they were. Exercise and general mobility will keep this under control to an extent, but the muscles will not return to normal until the inflammation has settled down almost completely. Do not get too troubled, therefore, if your arms and legs look rather spindly. When the arthritis settles the muscles will return to normal, but until then the best you can do is to keep them as mobile and supple as you can.

The purpose of any exercise is to put each joint through its own natural movements but not to subject it to any abnormal strains or contortions. Some joints, such as the knees only have one direction in which they move, while others, such as the wrist, can be moved in several, and your exercises should aim to reproduce these natural movements. As well as keeping the joints as supple as possible the exercises can be used as measures of progress as you will be able to see day by day whether your range of movement and degree of pain are worsening or improving.

The exercises given here are mainly the simplest and most basic way of practising the normal movements of each of the joints in the body without making them bear too much weight. All of them should be done slowly and you should not attempt to do any which are obviously too demanding for your own particular condition.

Feet and ankles

Lie down with your legs outstretched. Curl your toes as tightly as you can, then uncurl them again and rest.

To exercise your ankles, lie with your knee still and your heel resting on the ground or bed and move your toes round in a circle, first clockwise and then anti-clockwise. If you have someone there to help you he or she can rest a hand on your knee while you do it to keep your leg steady.

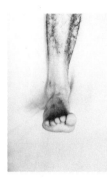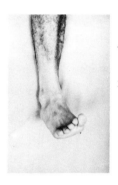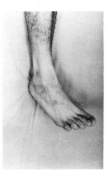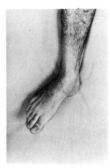

Knees

Exercise bicycles for use indoors are useful for maintaining knee movements and building up muscle tone in the legs. However even without such special apparatus you can get benefit from lying on your back and doing cycling movements in the air for two or three minutes. Two slightly less strenuous knee exercises you can do are as follows:

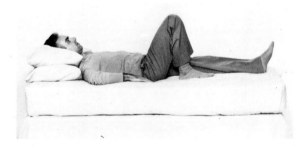

1. Lie on your back and slowly bend up one knee as far as it will go, then stretch the leg out straight again. Then do the same with your other leg and repeat the exercise several times.

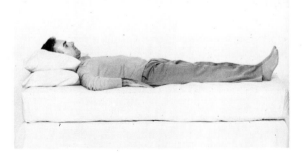

71

2. Lie straight with your feet pointing upwards. Slowly lift one leg (not necessarily very high, but just so that it is not touching the bed) keeping your knee straight and your thigh muscles braced. Lower it again slowly until the calf touches the bed and then relax. Again, do the exercise with each leg in turn.

Hips

The important thing with the hip is to rotate the joint so that the capsule around it does not contract or 'knit up'. A good exercise to help this is to lie on your back and slowly bend up both your legs. Separate your knees as wide apart as you can but keeping your heels together, and then close them back together again. Finally stretch out first one leg and then the other so that you are lying down straight as you were at the beginning.

Another hip exercise also begins in this position, lying on your back with your legs outstretched. One leg at a time, and keeping your knees straight, you lift your leg just clear of the bed, move it slowly out to the side as far as you can and then return it to its original position. Do these exercises several times until the joints begin to feel freer.

If your hips are stiff these movements will of course be restricted, but practising regularly will produce results as your range of movement gradually gets wider and less painful.

Loosening your hips:
1. Bring your knees up . . .   2. and out . . .

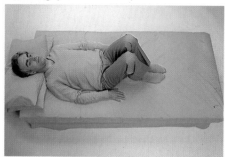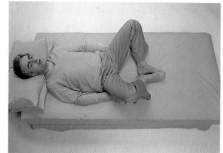

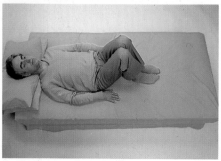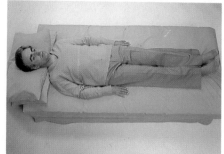

3. then together again.   4. Straighten each leg in turn.

Scissors exercise: 1. Lie flat.

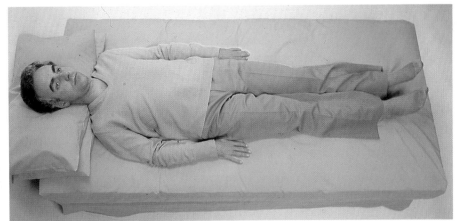

2. Lift your leg up off the bed . . .

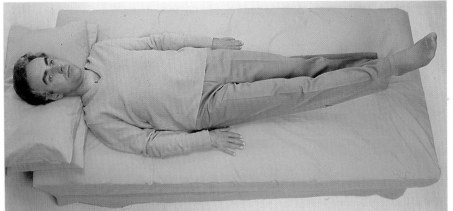

3. and take it out to the side. Then repeat the exercise with the other leg.

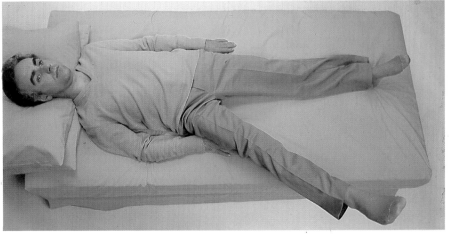

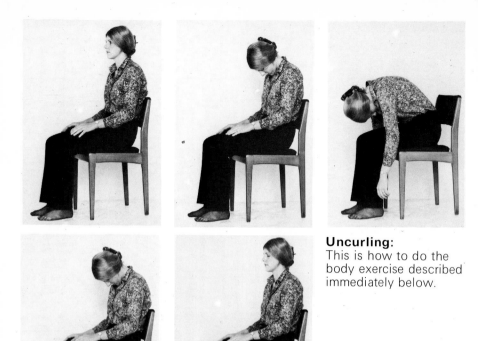

Uncurling:
This is how to do the
body exercise described
immediately below.

Body

Sit comfortably in a chair. Drop your head forward so that it touches your chest. Then gradually lean downwards towards your knees. Straighten up again, not unwinding your head until last.

Spine

The three movements of your spine which you should practise (unless your back is too acutely painful to make it possible) are bending backwards and forwards, bending sideways and turning to left and right. These exercises will put the spine through each of those movements:

1. Stand up and bend forwards towards your toes as far as you can. Then straighten up and, folding your arms across your chest, lean backwards so that you are looking towards the ceiling. Then bend forwards again. The exercise should be done as a gentle, continuous curling, starting at the base of the spine and working upward. It can also be done while lying down.

2. Stand up straight and then bend slowly sideways, running your left hand down your left thigh. Then straighten up again and do the same to the right.

3. Put your hands on your hips and rotate your spine so that, without moving your feet, you turn first to face the right and then to the left.

Shoulder and neck

These are two simple exercises for easing pain in the area of the neck and shoulders. The first is a movement which often comes naturally to anyone whose shoulders are feeling stiff after a day leaning over a desk or doing any tiring work. You start by shrugging your shoulders up as high as they will go. Then pull them right back, moving your shoulder blades closer towards each other, and then gradually relax them and bring them back down to a normal position.

Another good exercise is simply to clasp your hands together, first in front of you and then behind your back, repeating the movement several times.

The neck can be exercised by turning your head through its full range of movement, both left and right and up and down several times.

Elbows, wrists and hands

It is best to do these exercises with one arm at a time so that you can concentrate on that one, otherwise you will tend to find that whichever arm is the strongest ends up doing the most work.

The elbow's main movement is that of bending and stretching, so exercising this is simply a matter of sitting comfortably and bending and straightening your arm slowly as far as it will go in each direction.

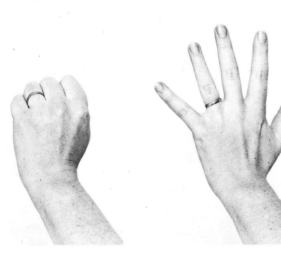

A good exercise for your hands is simply to clench them tightly and then spread out the fingers as widely as you can.

The best wrist exercise is to rotate each wrist right round. Sit with your elbows tucked in to your sides and move each hand in a complete circle, first in one direction and then in the other.

To exercise your hands as fully as possible you should try regularly squeezing them into a tight fist and then slowly stretching out your fingers as wide as possible, separating them from each other and then bringing them together again.

One exercise which, if you can complete it, will show that most of the joints in your arm are supple is the following. You begin by raising your arms above your head with the hands pressed flat against each other, palm to palm. Then, keeping the hands pressed together, you gradually bend your elbows and bring your hands down to your chest until your fingertips are just below your chin. Then rotate your wrists forwards until your fingers are pointing downwards. This is, of course, an ambitious exercise which involves a number of different movements in each joint and will only be possible for people whose arms and shoulders are very mobile.

Exercises in water (hydrotherapy)

Muscular movements and body exercises in water are of enormous help to many rheumatic sufferers as movements which are otherwise difficult or impossible can be done much more easily if the body is supported in water. In your own bath you can get the warming and relaxing effect of the water on your muscles and joints but can only make restricted movements. For full exercise you need to go to a swimming bath or pool provided it is one where the water is kept sufficiently warm. It will probably be helpful to take a friend with you who can assist you in and out of the pool and give you moral and physical support while doing the exercises.

Almost any activity in water will help stiff muscles and joints to function better, whether you swim gently using breast stroke, or float on your back or just stand at the edge of the pool with the water up to your neck and gradually put each of your joints in turn through its natural range of movements. Many of the exercises described in the previous section can be done much more easily in warm water. Some people find that a movement, let us say of the shoulders, which was perhaps only half normal when practised in the bedroom, can be raised almost to its complete range after a few sessions in the swimming bath.

In most physiotherapy centres the deep pool, if it exists, is the most popular part of the establishment with most of the patients. Many of them suffer from too severe an arthritis to be able to use a public pool but find

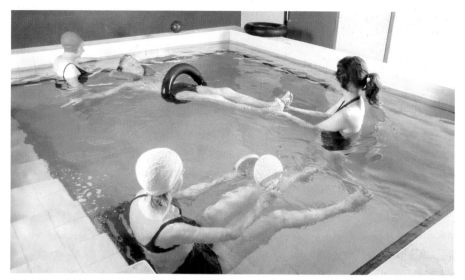

A hydrotherapy pool: The water in the pool is kept at about body temperature and enables patients to move through a greater range of movement with less pain. Movements out of the water should also improve as a result.

that exercising in warm water is good both for their joints and their morale. Unfortunately we do need many more of these special pools than are at present available.

Rest

The importance of resting your joints cannot be exaggerated. It is an essential part of the treatment for any inflamed or recently injured joint or if you have an acute back or neck ache. No one would attempt to walk a long way home on a broken leg or sprained ankle, and an arthritic joint should be treated with the same care. Rest is as much a part of pain relief as are warmth or analgesic pills.

Putting on a splint is a form of local rest and firm, cold compresses can also be used both to rest a damaged joint and to relieve the pain and swelling.

However, too much rest can harm your joints and if you have to lie in bed for long periods without moving your limbs, you should start gentle exercises as soon as the worst of the pain wears off. You may need a cradle to lift the bedclothes off your legs in order to be able to move more freely. Another good idea if you have to lie in bed for several weeks is to put a firm board or piece of cardboard across the mattress at the bottom of the bed to support your ankles and prevent your feet from dropping. You can exercise your feet by pushing against the board and then lifting and lowering them — a kind of walking exercise in bed!

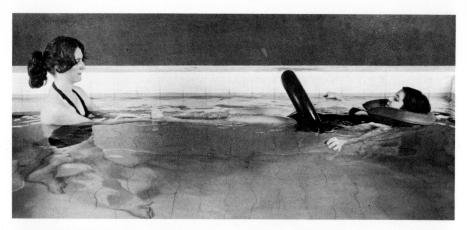

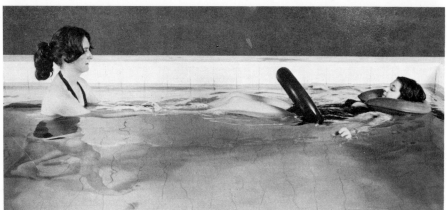

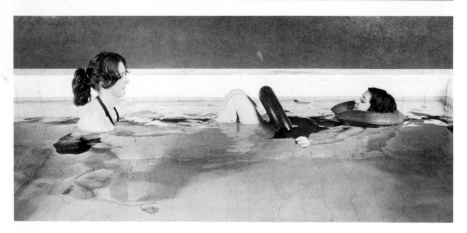

This demonstrates an exercise in water designed to improve movement after a hip operation. A physiotherapist ensures that the joint movements are correctly controlled, making use of the warmth, support and buoyancy of the water.

Relaxation

Muscles which are held constantly taut may become tender and there is no doubt that muscle tension plays a part in aggravating the aches and pains of many rheumatic disorders. It is therefore important not only to exercise and use the muscles positively, but also to have periods of relaxation when all the muscles are completely relaxed and your mind is at ease.

One of the most difficult things for most people to do is to relax properly. Quite a good plan is the following. Set aside a time each day when you will be left completely undisturbed for perhaps half an hour. Settle yourself somewhere where you can loosen your clothing and sit or lie completely relaxed. It is easier to relax the body than the mind so it may take several sessions before you get into the habit of relaxing completely mentally as well as bodily. Many books have been written on the gentle art of relaxation (including another book in this series, written by Jane Madders). In the rheumatic disorders this must be accompanied by a philosophy adapted to the rheumatic condition that one has. There is inestimable value in learning gradually to accept the situation, and get on with the practical art of living with your disability. You should fight it, certainly, with all the weapons at your disposal but aim not to fight yourself in the process.

Heat treatment

Heat is not magic and it will not cure arthritis although it does increase the local circulation to the joint and relieve some of the pain. Its main value, however, is that it is easier and less painful to exercise an arthritic joint when it is warmed. The routine you should follow, therefore, whatever form of heat treatment you use, should be: heat first, exercise second.

There is no particular virtue in any one form of heat over another and hot pads or warm bandages, dry or wet (the so-called old-fashioned hot stupes) can all be applied to the suffering area equally effectively. You can also buy specially made electrically heated pads to put round the area of pain (see page 81). When the joint is gently glowing it should be exercised. Some patients prefer cold applications such as ice packs or cold sprays. (It is important to remember that ice must not be applied directly to the skin, but should be put in a bag or other container.) Like heat these leave a pleasant afterglow and induce a phase of increased circulation while you do your exercises, but most people seem to prefer heat treatments.

A hot bath or shower is the best and simplest form of providing heat in your home, but any safe and well-designed lamp or electric heater can also be used, as long as you take great care to avoid over-exposure, as burns from these lamps can be most unpleasant.

If your hands or wrists are affected, a good treatment is to bathe them in hot water until they are gently glowing and then squeeze a sponge or other soft object gently several times. Then take your hands out of the water and do, as it were, piano playing exercises on the edge of the basin – moving your fingers and wrists in all directions. The same routine of hot water soaks followed by exercises can be applied to toes, feet and ankles. Such exercises are as good in many cases as hot wax applications and less dangerous, as wax may sometimes catch fire.

Some people do get relief from applying special low melting-point wax to their hands (usually by painting it on with a brush), then enclosing them in a warm towel for a while before removing the wax and doing gentle exercises. However I would always recommend hot water as the preferable alternative. It is easier, cheaper, less hazardous and generally just as effective.

Rubs

Various liniments, creams, embrocations and ointments ('rubs') are a way in which patients can give themselves their own massage and counter-irritation, or can ask their husbands and wives to do it for them. Most rubs act by causing a mild inflammation and irritation of the skin which increases the circulation to the area slightly and applies gentle massage at the same time. This, again, is a form of heat and should be followed by exercise.

There is no great virtue of one rub over another. Some have a more, some a less strong effect and you should beware of over-using the more powerful varieties as they can cause skin burns. In almost all cases the effect is a purely local one, easing the pain in the area to which it is applied. Massaging should always be done in firm strokes with the flat palm of the hand rather than with the finger tips.

Surgery

There are a number of operations which can be done to give considerable help to people suffering from severe arthritis. Of the major ones the hip replacement is perhaps the most dramatically effective. This involves removing the entire hip and replacing it with a false joint. It is obviously quite a major operation and is therefore only carried out when patients are in such constant or intolerable pain that life with the hip nature gave them has become almost unliveable. The results of the operation, however,

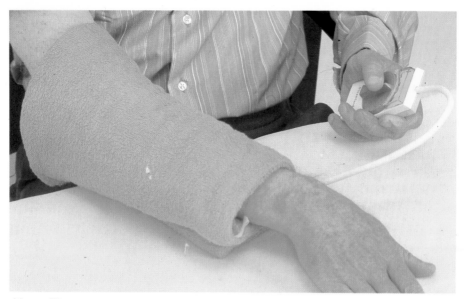

Above There are many ways of applying warmth to your joints. One method is to use a special electric heating pad such as this one, which is controlled by a hand-held thermostat.

Below While heating your hands in a bowl of warm water you can exercise them by squeezing a sponge, and then gently drumming your fingers on the table.

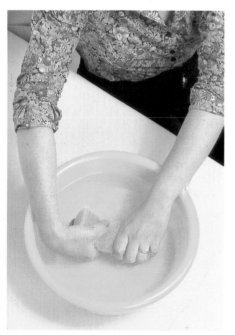
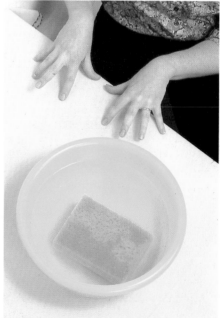

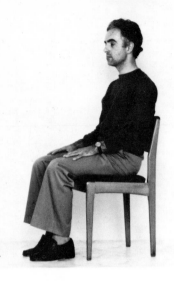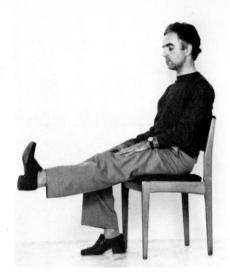

Strengthening the thigh muscles:
1. Sit with your feet flat on the ground. 2. Raise your leg straight out in front of you and then slowly lower it again.

have been known to make a truly spectacular difference both in relieving the agonising pain and in restoring the patient's mobility.

Most people are discharged from hospital as little as two weeks after the operation, during which time they have progressed from walking with elbow crutches to needing only sticks. By around the twelfth day they can usually go up and down stairs and sit without pain in ordinary chairs.

You will need individual advice on the kinds of exercise which you should or should not do after your own particular operation as you gradually build up strength and increase your range. Walking and swimming are both good in most instances, and it is always important to do all you can to strengthen your thigh muscles. An easy exercise for doing this is simply to sit in a chair and lift and straighten each leg in turn several times.

There are many other more minor operations which will help correct such things as deformed and painful toes, severe rheumatoid wrists or ruptured tendons and all of these usually give excellent results.

Manipulation

There is no doubt that many chronic pains, particularly back ache, can be greatly helped by an expert manipulator. Any weight-bearing joints such as knees and hips which have been affected by osteo-arthrosis and which have not responded to other kinds of therapy may also be helped by manipulation, but there is little place for it in inflammatory disorders such as rheumatoid arthritis except sometimes in the later stages, but even then it is a risk as rheumatoid tissues can be all too readily damaged. Patients with ankylosing spondylitis should not in general be manipulated as it often makes them feel worse rather than better.

Manipulation can sometimes be dramatically effective in relieving acute symptoms, but it tends to be a matter of chance. As with shuffling a pack of cards, the ace may come up or it may not, and results may be good, bad or indifferent depending on the state of the disease and the expertise of the manipulator. And even in the best hands this treatment is always something of a gamble as no one can predict the results with absolute certainty.

Acupuncture

This ancient Chinese form of therapy can produce definite pain relief, particularly in cases of chronic osteo-arthrosis and soft tissue rheumatism. It is done by a complex system of placing needles in specific parts of the body believed to be in some way related to the afflicted areas. It does not cure the underlying disease but it can nonetheless be successful in easing the pain and, if it works for you, you can go back for extra sessions if and when your arthritis starts to get worse again.

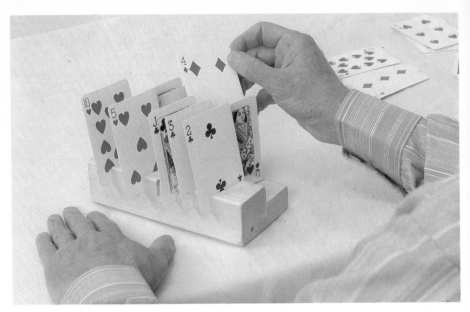

Holding a fan of playing cards can be awkward and bad for arthritic hands. This simple wooden holder does the job for you.

Long-handled dustpans and brooms can spare you much of the painful bending involved in doing the housework.

A push button telephone is easier on the fingers than one with a dial.

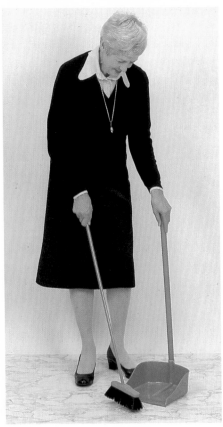

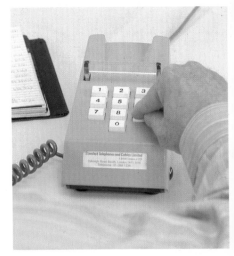

6. COPING WITH ARTHRITIS IN EVERYDAY LIFE

Adapting your home

In fighting any war you have to use your wits as well as all the weapons available, and there are lots of good ideas and helpful gadgets around to combat the difficulties of living with a disability. The Arthritis and Rheumatism Council put out an excellent small book entitled 'Your Home and Your Rheumatism' and what I am going to say here comes very largely from this. It is not impossible to have an ideal home planned to take care of all your rheumatic troubles and, depending on your type of arthritis and the joints involved, there are a number of special devices you can buy and minor adaptations you can make to your environment which could make all the difference to your daily comfort and progress.

Aids and tips

Electric points throughout the house are sometimes inaccessible and raising the sockets higher up the wall to about waist height may be a great help, although it is of course a considerable undertaking. Electric light switches can be specially adapted for arthritic fingers and in some cases pull cords hanging from the ceiling are easier to manage than switches.

Be careful over floor surfaces. Small mats can be dangerous as they may slip on the polished floor beneath. Many a bone has been broken as a result of this. Beware also of holes in carpets, torn pieces of linoleum and any other potential hazards. One of the worst things that can happen to an elderly arthritic sufferer is to fall and fracture a leg after tripping over some such trap. Elderly people do not recover lightly after an accident like this, particularly if they fracture their femur (thigh bone).

Door knobs are very difficult for many arthritics and a lever type handle is generally better than the ordinary kind of door knob as it can be moved with the elbow or forearm instead of the hand. A push button telephone is easier to manage then the type where you have to put your finger into holes in the dial. One of the most useful gadgets in the home is the so-called 'helping hand' or 'lazy tongs' illustrated on page 87. It can pick things up from the floor or table and has a small magnet in the end for picking up pins or other metal objects.

If you find it difficult to bend down and pick up letters in the hall, a

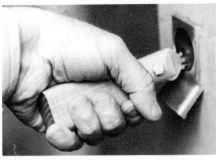

Keys are less trouble to grip and turn if you mount them on a thick wooden handle.

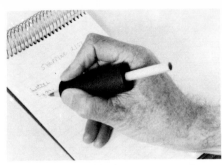

A piece of thickening put round a pen enlarges the grip and so can make writing much less difficult.

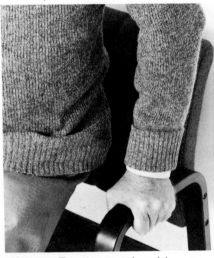

Wrong: Try not to grip with your hands when getting out of a chair.

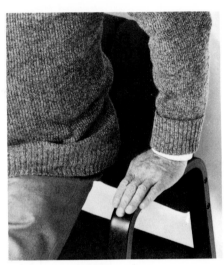

Right: It is better to keep your hands flat like this.

Above Right Helping hand tongs can be useful for many tasks about the house, and save a lot of unnecessary bending or stretching.

Right Raising the height of your chair legs with blocks, or specially made sleeves like these, may make it easier for you to get in and out of it. When sitting in a raised chair you will probably find it comfortable to rest your feet on a footstool.

Far Right This spring-loaded 'ejector' seat helps with the problem of getting in and out of a low chair.

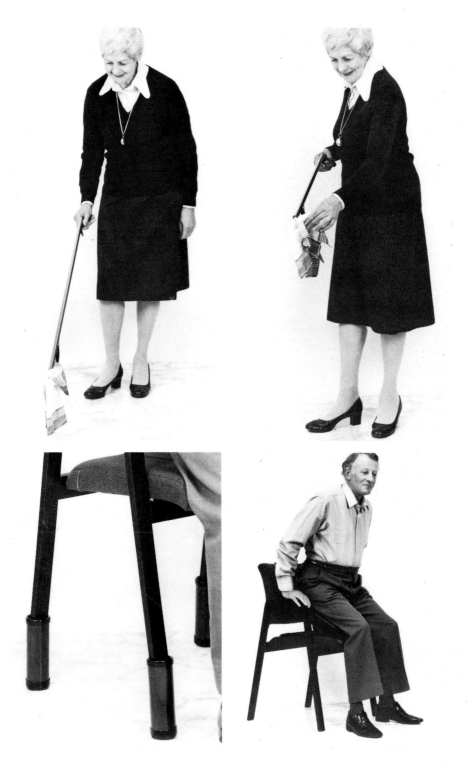

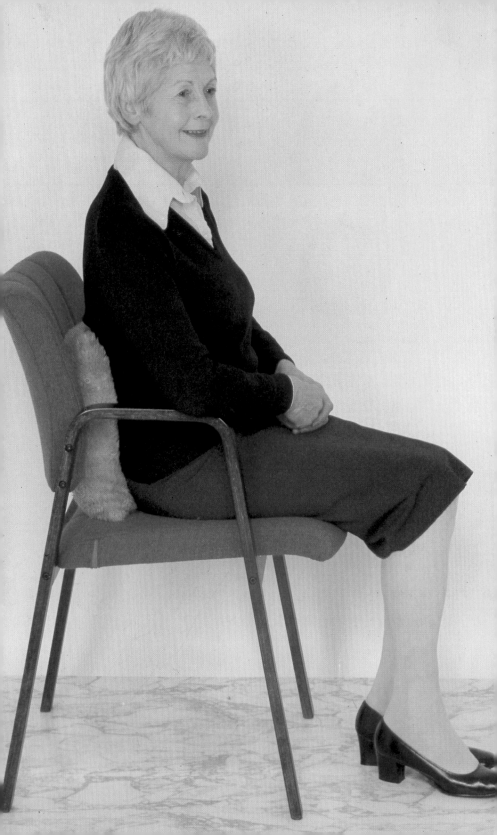

simple and useful solution to this problem is to fix up a wire basket to catch them before they drop to the ground.

Stairs

These can be a major difficulty and the ideal thing for a patient with acute arthritis is to live on one level, even if this means converting a downstairs room for the time being so that bed, lavatory and kitchen can all be together. If this is not possible you should at least, particularly if you have arthritic knees, try to go up and down stairs as seldom as possible.

You can fit special half stairs, which are small blocks of wood placed at the side of each step to make them half the normal height. Another idea is to make yourself a small portable step on a string or long handle. There are also special lifts, but these are an elaborate installation and only feasible for people who have enough money or expertise to make major adaptations to their homes.

Hand rails may be all that is needed in many cases, and it is best if possible to have one rail on each side of the staircase. There should be a non-slip finish to the treads as carpets can be dangerous if they are not securely fixed. Lighting is particularly important over stairs and landings. In poor light it is all too easy to trip and fall.

Chairs

The furniture used regularly in any room is always important and has to be designed very much to suit your own individual measurements and type of disability. You should have one particular chair in each room which you know you can sit in comfortably and which is of the right height with

Left Something as simple as putting a cushion behind your back can sometimes make all the difference to your comfort.

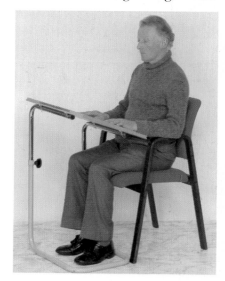

Right A tilting table can be adjusted to suit you and makes tasks such as reading and writing less troublesome.

a firm, supporting back and also, preferably, arm rests. Raising the height of the chair by lengthening the legs or putting blocks under them is sometimes necessary for patients with very stiff knees who just cannot get into or out of a low chair.

There are a number of special chairs with raised seats on the market, and also some with 'ejector seats' which allow you, as it were, to propel yourself mechanically from a sitting to a standing position. Putting a small cushion in the small of the back whenever you are sitting down for long periods can give great relief, particularly if you have back ache, and this is a useful tip not only in the house but also for when you have to travel by car or train.

Reading and writing

A simple tilting table is a useful aid to doing a number of tasks, including reading and writing. If it is fitted on large castors it can easily be pushed away without toppling. Some of these small tables on castors can be, and indeed often are, used by disabled patients as supports when they are walking from one room to another. The height of the chair in relation to the table is important as you should be able to work in a comfortable position. When writing at a table your spine should be firmly supported by the back of the chair and should be comfortably relaxed without being either slouched or stooping. Writing paper can be held steady by a magnetic board or by putting a bar across it which will keep it still. For patients with a poor grip, a felt thickening can be put around the pencil or pen so that it can be held more easily. There are quite a number of these available at occupational centres and hospitals.

For reading there are various simple bookstands which will hold a book in front of you so that you do not have to hold it in your hands, and some of the tilting tables I have already mentioned have adjustable rests for books. For a very disabled person it is possible to obtain an electric page turner, but this is an extreme measure and rarely necessary.

The kitchen

The most important thing about the design of a kitchen for an arthritic sufferer is that all the furniture should be at the right height. For instance, anyone with painful hips or knees who is unable to stand for prolonged periods, must have a high chair at the sink of the right height for washing up, and one adjusted to the height of the cooker so that the back is not bent and the shoulders and arms are comfortably above the level of the pots and pans. The chairs at a kitchen table should likewise allow you to do all the various kitchen chores without bending or stooping un-necessarily. In many cases only modest adaptations are required and these

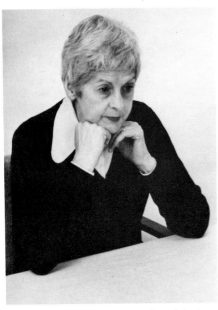

Wrong: It may feel comfortable but it is bad for arthritic hands to curl them under your chin like this.

Wrong: Holding heavy books puts a strain on the joints in your hands.

Right: Flat on the table is better.

Right: Buying or making a simple book rest such as this is the best solution to the problem.

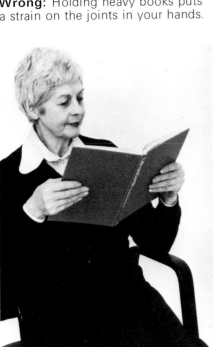

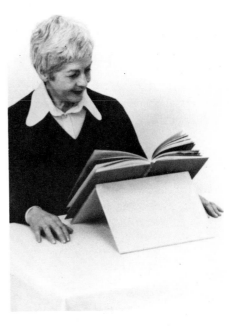

can be done by a local handyman. It is however wise to get some advice beforehand from a doctor, physiotherapist, occupational therapist or district nurse.

If everything is at the same height and without gaps between one surface and the next, heavy pans can be slid sideways instead of having to be lifted from one level to another.

Many of my patients prefer a shallow sink about 6 inches (0.2m) deep to the normal deeper kind. Lever taps which can be worked with the elbow, back of the hand or wrist are preferable to the usual screw taps, and if this is not practical a special tap turner can be used. Some water authorities are happy to modify the type and position of taps for you and this is worth checking. Swivel-type tap fitments, preferably fixed off centre, are extremely helpful as they allow you to fill kettles and saucepans without lifting them into and out of the sink.

There are also a number of modifications which can be made to the taps on gas and electric cookers. When choosing a new cooker it is desirable to find one in which the oven and burners are separate, so that the oven can be installed at waist or shoulder height. Alternatively there is a small and relatively inexpensive kind of oven which rests on top of the hot plates which might prove a good substitute.

The height of the refrigerator may need to be increased so that you don't have to bend down too frequently, and if you are buying a new one you might decide that a table or wall model would be easier to reach. Most new designs are easy to open and shut.

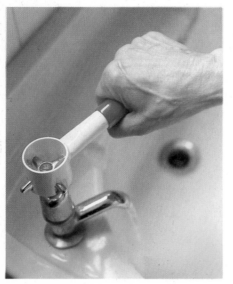

Left Turning taps in the bathroom or kitchen is easier with a long lever.

Right A supportive, raised chair like this in the kitchen could take much of the pain and effort out of the hours you spend at the sink or the cooker. You might be glad of a cushion to support your back.

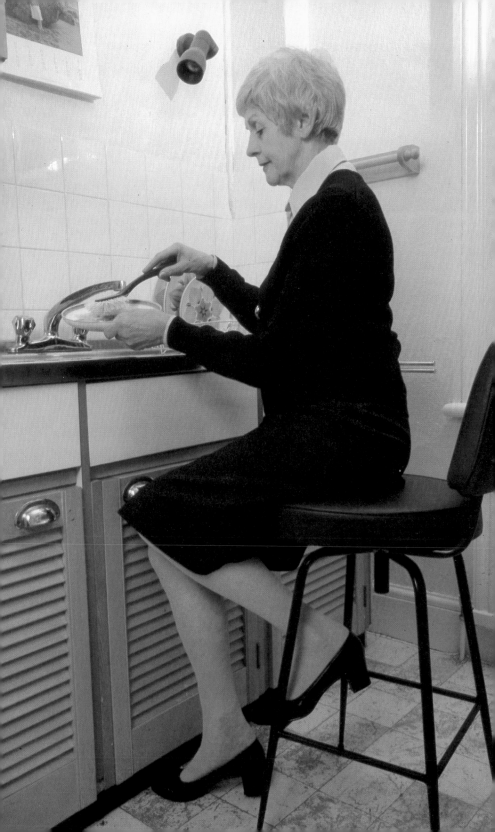

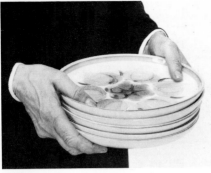

Wrong: Try to avoid carrying heavy weights with your hands gripped round them.

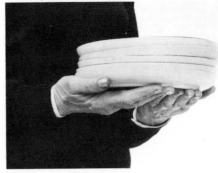

Right: Instead, if you can manage it comfortably, put your hands flat underneath, like this.

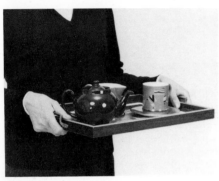

Wrong

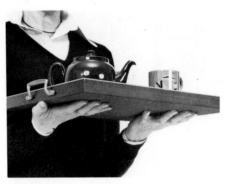

Right: The same goes for a tea tray. If your grip is weak it is safer as well as better for your hands to carry the tray like this.

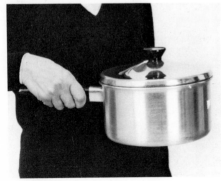

Wrong: Carrying a one-handled saucepan in the normal way can be difficult for arthritic hands.

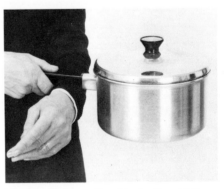

Right: This method is better. If the pan is hot you can protect your hands from burning with an overn cloth.

It is important for shelves and cupboards to be at a sensible height so that you can take food or utensils in and out without causing too much strain to your spine, elbow or shoulder. Sometimes you can fit sliding or rotating shelves. Drawers are best if they are shallow, and hold only one level of utensils. Sliding doors for wall units are sometimes easier to move than those with hinges. Saucepans need to be light and should have a heat-resistant handle on each side to make them easy to lift with two hands. Handles on pans and jars can be enlarged if necessary.

There are a larger number of aids available to help with preparing food. Knives and other cutlery are often easier to manage if a piece of felt or other form of thickening is fixed around their handles. Tools such as food crushers and special combined fork-cum-knives can sometimes be useful additions to the normal range of cutting implements. Vegetables can be held steady by being impaled on nails fixed into chopping boards. Alternatively a potato peeler can be fixed to the table so that you can use both hands to peel the vegetable. Some electric mixers also of course have a special attachment which will do your potato peeling automatically.

You can hold a mixing bowl still while making pastry or cakes by putting a damp cloth underneath it or by using a variety of specially designed suction or wooden attachments. For whisking there are

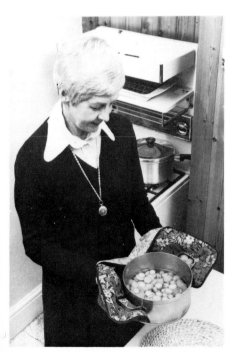

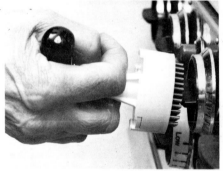

Above There are several gadgets available to help if you have trouble adjusting the knobs on your cooker. This one has a clump of retractable pins which grip the knob firmly while you turn, and it can be used equally well on any small, fiddly knobs and taps about the house.

Left Saucepans with two handles are easier because you can spread the load.

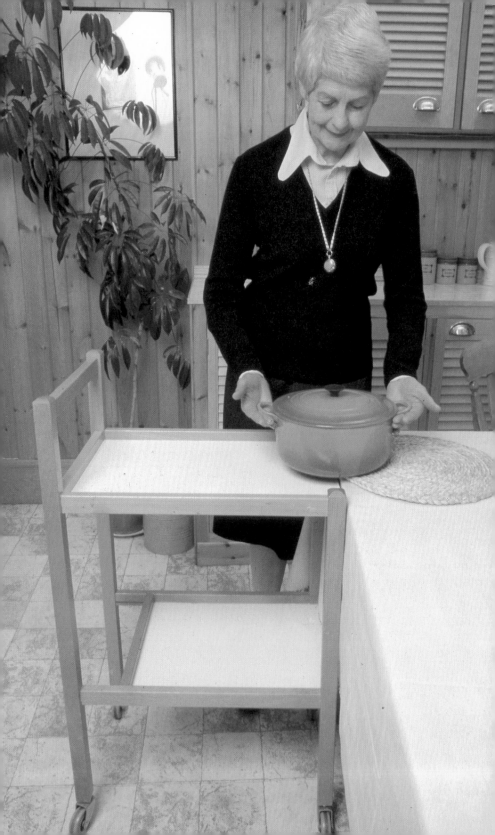

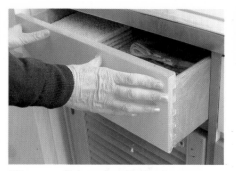
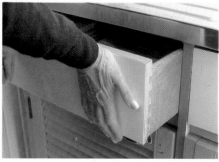

Wrong: This way of shutting a drawer is bad for your hands.

Right: Keeping them flat like this is better.

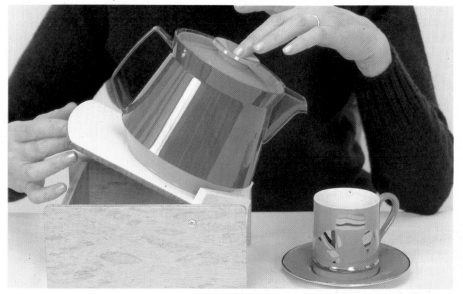

Above A special tipper like this makes pouring tea out of a heavy pot much easier.

Right Peeling potatoes with an ordinary peeler is often painful and difficult for arthritic hands. A peeler that can be clamped to the table like this makes the task less arduous.

Left A trolley at the same height as your kitchen surfaces can save you a lot of lifting and carrying.

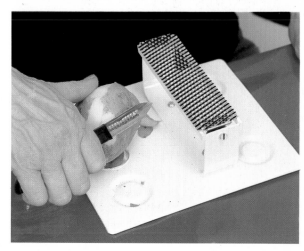

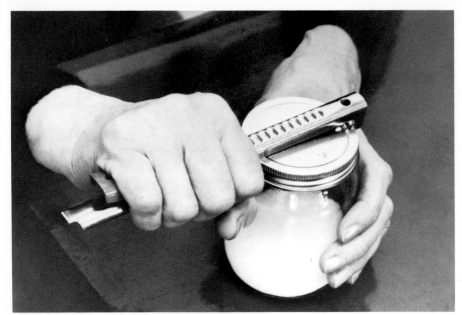

This is just one of the many gadgets around to help with the difficult task of opening jars.

Lifting vegetables out of a pan with a chip basket is lighter and safer than carrying the hot, laden pan across the kitchen.

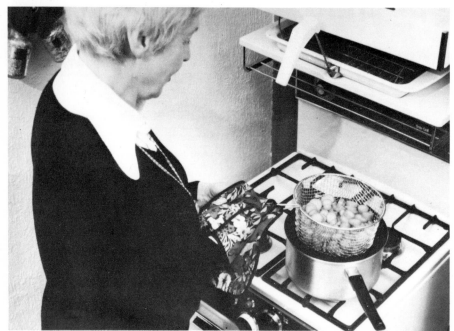

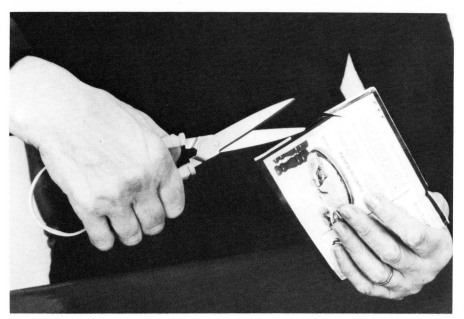

If you find ordinary scissors hard to use, this type which you simply squeeze might solve the problem.

numerous types of light egg whisk obtainable which can be used with one hand. There is also on the market an invaluable special opener which binds tightly around a jar or bottle and can then be worked with relative ease to unscrew a stiff top. For opening tins the best thing is a tin opener fixed to the wall which can be adjusted for different sizes of tin. Another useful little gadget is a teapot tipper which will spare you the effort of lifting a heavy pot up in order to pour out the tea.

A trolley is another very useful piece of kitchen equipment, made at the right height to allow you to wheel it without discomfort and so that heavy objects can be slid onto it from other kitchen surfaces and transported without any lifting at all.

The bathroom

Perhaps the most difficult rooms in the house, and sometimes almost torture chambers, for the arthritic sufferer are the bathroom and lavatory. The first expedition to the bathroom after the onset of rheumatoid arthritis can be a traumatic experience, and the patient may greatly appreciate the assistance of a friend, relative or nurse on this occasion.

Many people with arthritis are unable to manage an ordinary bath and may well strain their joints trying to get in and out of it. Some develop a technique of getting out by sliding onto their side and then into a kneeling

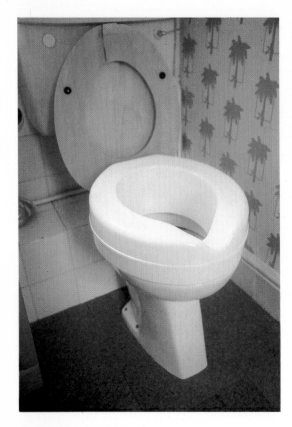

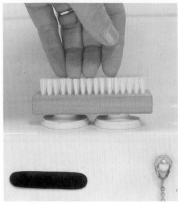

Above A nail brush with suction pads means you do not need to hold it while you scrub your nails.

Left Fitting a raised lavatory seat is a good idea for anyone with stiff hips.

position before finally rising, but the whole manoeuvre is quite an ordeal. A shower is often a better idea, and it can either be fitted in its own compartment or attached to the taps of the bath.

Steps may be necessary to help you get in and out of the bath, and, once in, a non-slip rubber mat or even a small seat could make bathing easier. If you have severely limited movement in your knees or hips an over-bath seat or board extending across the bath onto the floor or with a stool the same height may be necessary.

The bedroom

The height and design of your bed can make an important difference not only to your comfort at night but also to how stiff you will feel the next day. The bed should not be too high and it should be firm enough to support your spine comfortably and gently but without sagging. If you have chronic back ache it is usually essential to put a board under the mattress to keep your spine straight while sleeping. You may find it more comfortable if you have two mattresses on top of the board to take some of the hardness out.

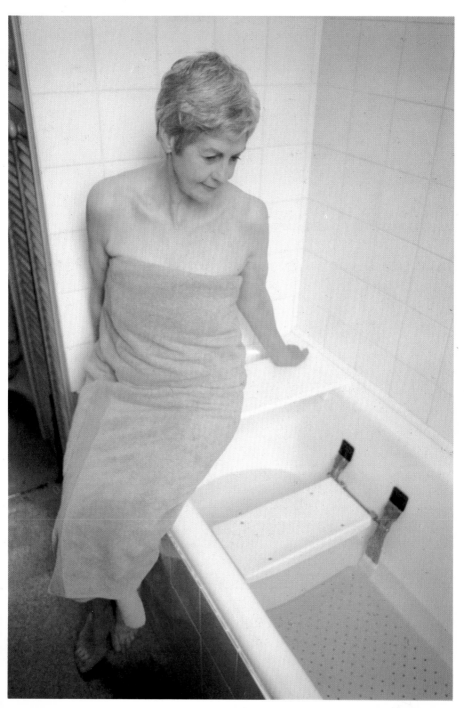

A board fixed across the bath can be a great help when getting in and out. A bath seat and a non-slip mat are also a good idea.

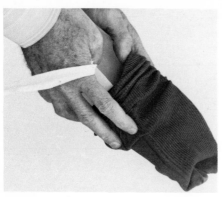

A stocking aid. Fix the sock or stocking round the flexible piece of plastic. Then you can use the tapes to pull it on without having to bend down.

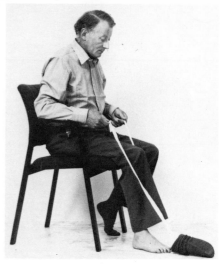

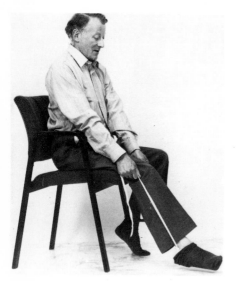

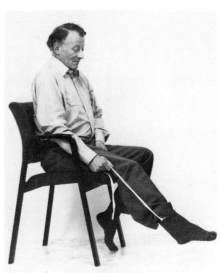

Double beds may be a source of considerable unhappiness, as a bed which is comfortable for a normal person is often totally unsuitable for someone suffering from arthritis. It is probably better to arrange two single beds alongside each other than to force the poor arthritic sufferer to sleep in a type of bed that is unsuitable for his or her damaged joints.

Tightly tucked in bedclothes are difficult or impossible for many rheumatoid sufferers with weak wrists and hands. Loose fitting blankets and sheets are better, and perhaps best of all is a continental quilt or duvet which is light and can be easily moved while still providing a good warm covering.

Warmth in bed is important. Bed socks are a good way to keep your feet warm and electric blankets can help warm the bed before you get in, but should never be left switched on when you go to sleep. Similarly it can be a good idea to heat up your nightwear and the bed with hot water bottles, but you should not go to sleep with a hot bottle pressed against your skin as many burns have occurred in this way and rheumatoid sufferers in particular find that any such burns or damage to the skin tend to heal more slowly than they do with other people.

Many patients evolve their own devices for getting dressed and undressed, but a visit to an occupational centre or specialist shop might give you some good new ideas. There are lots of devices available such as a gadget for pulling up socks and stockings, a long-handled shoe horn and a special tool to help people with painful shoulders comb their hair. If you have arthritic hands it may be a good idea to sew extra-large buttons onto your clothes and to use a special button hook to do them up and undo them.

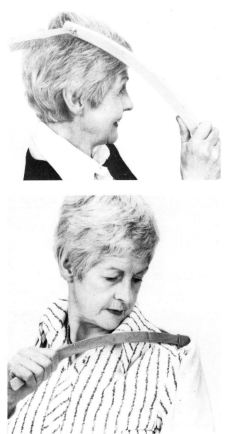

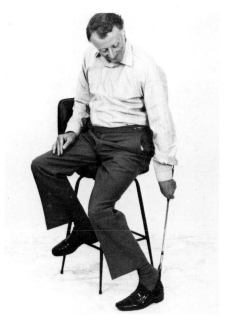

Above Left A long-handled comb.

Left A simple dressing stick takes some of the effort out of getting clothes on or off.

Above A shoe horn with an extra-long handle.

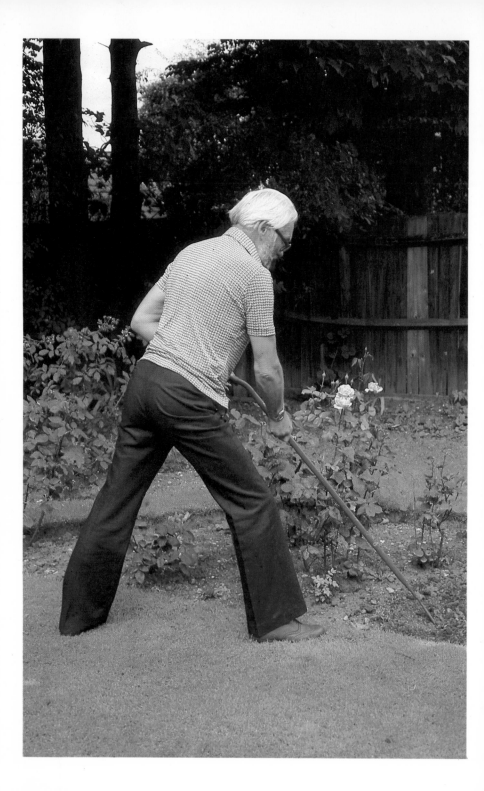

Gardening

Working in the garden can be a very relaxing hobby. It can soothe the nerves and give you all the benefits of fresh air and exercise. It can also aggravate almost every joint in your body if it is done too vigorously. At the first sign of spring the amateur gardener tends to rush into the garden and with high enthusiasm does many things he or she would not normally think of doing, and later suffers terrible pains in the joints accordingly.

Crouching over the ground with the knees flexed and back bent may aggravate knees, ankle and spine and although probably no lasting damage is done, aches from these areas can persist for several days or weeks. It is best to kneel on rubber pads and keep the spine as straight as possible, or to lean well forward with one hand on the ground and do any weeding or planting with the other. Special long handled gardening tools or the well tried device of building raised flower beds in your garden will both spare you some of the pain and effort of bending down for long periods.

Lifting wheelbarrows, mowing the lawn or digging in heavy soil may also cause an aggravation of a back ache long forgotten. It is best to garden as the professionals do, gently, not too fast and with a conservation of energy. Enthusiasm in the garden is a good thing but over-enthusiasm or too aggressive an approach will do your arthritis no good at all. You may be, in the poet's words 'nearer to God in a garden than anywhere else on earth', but one might truthfully add that the pains and aches you get tend to be diabolical rather than celestial.

Left Long handled tools take some of the strain out of gardening.

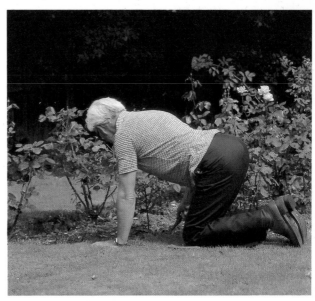

Right Kneeling on a pad with your spine straight is the best way to do the weeding.

Your arthritis and your car

If you have arthritis you may well be particularly dependent on your car for the added mobility it gives you. When choosing which car to buy, people with stiff hips, knees or hands should make a point of getting in and out of the car several times to check that the design suits their own disability. Each case will of course have individual problems and requirements but here are some of the general points you should watch out for:

1. The height of the car seat above the ground or kerb.

2. The width of the door.

3. The space between the door, when open, and the front of the driving seat.

4. How easy it is to get in from the passenger side and then move across into the driving seat. (This can be particularly important if you are parked in a busy road and need plenty of time to get yourself comfortably settled in the car.)

5. The positioning of the steering wheel and other controls, which can sometimes make getting in and out unnecessarily difficult.

6. The height between the seat and the top of the door. Extended runners which allow the seat to run backwards further than normal can give useful extra swing-in space for people with stiff knees. Fully adjustable swivelling seats are also available.

Check that the positioning of the seat and controls is reasonable for you. You should be able to drive comfortably with your knees slightly bent. The design of the seat itself is also important so that your back will be well supported and not slouched. You can if necessary buy a plastic support which will clip over the seat, or you can arrange pillows in the small of your back to make it more comfortable.

Light steering is often important to arthritic drivers and this is something you should test when the car is moving at slow speeds. It is possible to get power assisted steering, although this is usually only available as an option on heavier cars. If you want it fitted you should make sure you have it done before delivery of a new car, as it is expensive to have it converted later.

Automatic gears can of course be a great boon in taking some of the effort out of driving. They are a more expensive investment than manual ones but will remain an asset when you sell the car and, if you want to do a conversion to hand controls, this is simpler with an automatic car.

106

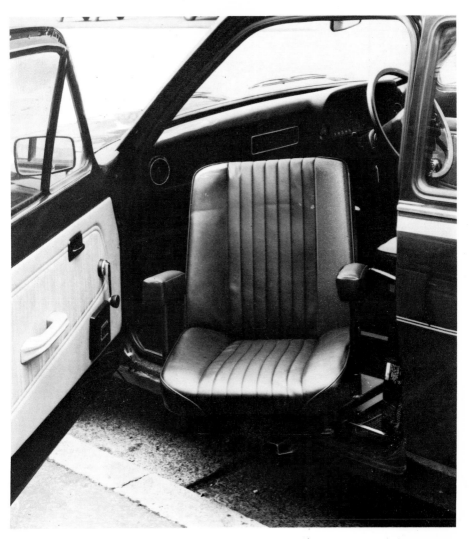

A swivelling seat which can be simply fitted and will save much of the strain of getting in and out of the car.

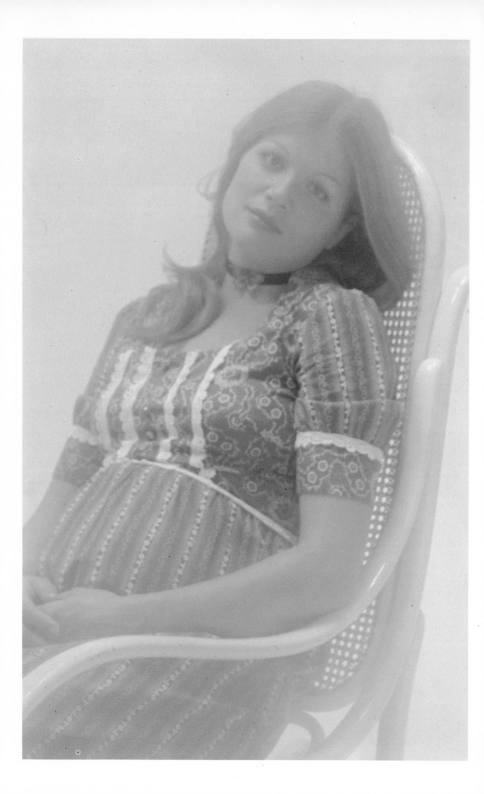

Sex

In many cases arthritis can have a major effect on married life. If it affects the hips, spine and knees it may make love-making extremely painful and very often indeed lead to a complete cessation of sexual relations. This is often simply due to the pain itself, but the illness that goes with it, particularly in the case of rheumatoid arthritis, may also diminish the sex urge quite considerably.

There is, however, no doubt that the damage caused to matrimonial relationships by arthritis could often be avoided by a few simple modifications to the sex act. A woman who is unable, because of arthritis, to rotate her hips or spread her legs is in some cases unable to make love at all unless she and her partner can experiment with different positions and find one which is acceptable to both. Because arthritic sufferers very often have a diminished sexual desire they may need more love play and caressing before they are ready for intercourse.

Many of the surgical operations done on the hips in the old days used to make it impossible for the patient to have sex thereafter, but more modern operations which involve the replacement of the hip joint very often restore normal sexual relations for patients who, before the operation, were in too much pain to enjoy making love.

Love, affection and mutual esteem between married people is more a spiritual than a physical thing, but if the physical expression of love is made impossible or painful this can understandably have an adverse effect on the marriage. Chronic arthritis makes great demands not only on the patient but also on his or her partner, and mutual sympathy and help are especially important in a marriage where one person is ill or disabled.

Pregnancy

There is rarely any good reason why a woman should be deterred from having children just because she has an arthritic condition, as all the chances are that she will have a successful pregnancy and childbirth, and that the baby will be born completely normal. There will of course be some added difficulties for the mother with arthritis and she will probably find the hard work of looking after a new baby much more of a struggle, but this is a problem most couples seem well ready to face in return for the rewards of bringing up a family.

Low back pain is common during pregnancy and often lasts for some time even after the birth. Some women worry that these pains may be signs of the onset of arthritis, but this is highly unlikely. Any pre-natal clinic will give advice on exercises which will help the pains, and the exercises you do after the baby has been born in order to tighten up the tummy muscles will also relieve some of the back ache.

Osteo-arthrosis does not usually develop until after childbearing age, but occasionally young women may, for example, get an osteo-arthritic hip as a result of an injury. Childbearing can be quite normal when one hip is stiff and painful, and even if both hips are affected there should not be any insurmountable problems in delivering the child safely although in this case a Caesarian section will probably be necessary.

Rheumatoid arthritis tends, in 75 per cent of cases, actually to improve during pregnancy. Most mothers find that their symptoms settle down or completely disappear throughout the period when they are carrying the baby, although the disease generally worsens again immediately after the birth. This of course is just the time when the young mother will be faced with new and additional work looking after her child, and she may need special reserves of mental strength to cope with the return of her arthritis after the respite she enjoyed during her pregnancy.

There is very little evidence to suggest that anti-rheumatic drugs can affect an unborn child, but if your rheumatoid arthritis does not follow the normal pattern and get better during pregnancy, allowing you to give up taking the drugs, you would still be well advised to consult your doctor just to make absolutely sure that any medicines you do continue taking are safe for the child.

A great deal of research has been done into why rheumatoid arthritis should improve during pregnancy and this may one day provide a clue as to how to cure the disease, although so far no one has come up with any really conclusive answers.

Whether you can cope with children will of course largely depend on what kind of arthritis you have got and how bad it is. In general, however, people with arthritis can rest assured that, if they want children and are confident that they will have the strength to look after them and bring them up, they need have no special reasons to be worried about getting pregnant.

Family relationships

A person who has any form of arthritis is likely to be disabled to some extent and therefore more dependent than most people on his or her relatives. Grandmother with osteo-arthrosis of her knees or hips will need helping up out of chairs and up or down stairs. Mother with rheumatoid arthritis may have to be assisted with the housekeeping or other daily tasks. Along with this physical assistance it is important for the family to

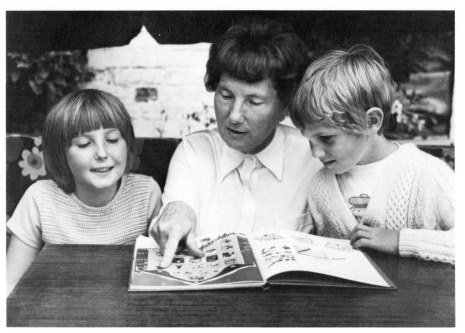

The support of a loving family can make the aches and pains of arthritits very much easier to bear.

provide what might be called SS and SS – silent sympathy and spiritual support – so that the unfortunate sufferer does not feel left alone in his or her battle against disability.

It is, however, necessary to achieve the right balance between too little help and too much. Many, and in my experience most, truly arthritic sufferers make few demands on their families. They prefer to struggle on as independently as possible and only ask for assistance when it is absolutely necessary. In some cases these stoics do not ask enough help and suffer needlessly as a result of performing painful duties that could well be done by someone else. Joints are meant to move and be used, but a severely diseased, painful, swollen or inflamed joint needs rest and a patient with a rheumatoid joint which has got worse as a result of doing specific domestic chores should pass those tasks on to another member of the family.

At the other extreme there are the over-complainers who, often with very little disability, make enormous demands on their families, and may suffer more themselves as a result. If they are given too much sympathy and assistance the patients end up doing too little and lose the will to keep going which is so essential for most arthritics. They become stiff and more incapacitated and therefore complain and lean more heavily on their families. This vicious circle must be corrected and the sufferers be

111

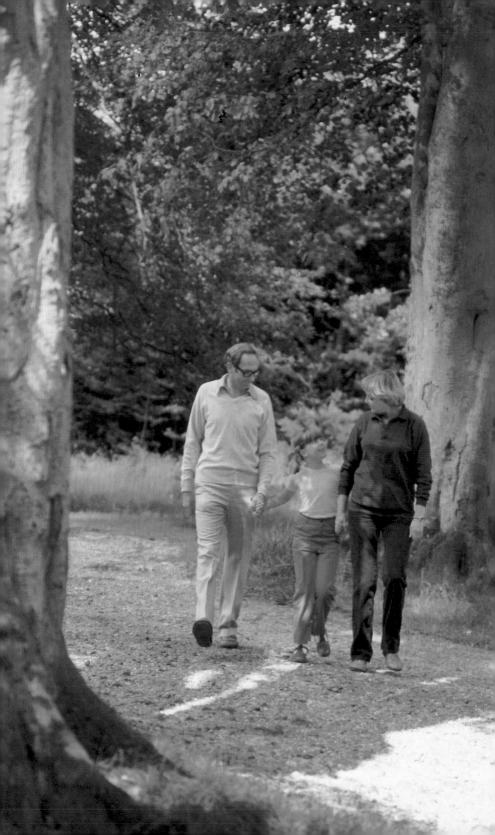

encouraged to do as much as possible for themselves.

Every family is unique in this respect and each individual case will depend on the disability and the character of the particular person involved and the attitude of those around him or her. The family should aim to encourage, provide sympathy and assist but not to take over their relative's arthritis altogether. Arthritis is in the end always a personal fight for whoever is afflicted with it, but the fight will be easier if practical assistance is available when required and SS and SS provided at all times.

There are of course people who have not got families around them to help and they need particular support from friends, neighbours and doctors. Arthritis and loneliness make an ugly combination. To be suffering pain, stiffness and disability without having anyone to turn to makes the whole disorder more depressing and harder to bear. Nevertheless, many gallant men and women living alone do manage to keep going in an extemely efficient way. Once again, if their attitude towards their arthritis is positive they can learn to be highly independent in spite of the burdens and limitations of their disability, and to face the future with exemplary courage and optimism.

USEFUL ADDRESSES

BRITAIN

The Arthritis and Rheumatism Council
Faraday House
8–10 Charing Cross Road
London WC2

The Arthritis and Rheumatism Council for Research and Education
41 Eagle Street
London WC1

The Back Pain Association
31–3 Park Road
Teddington
Middlesex

British League against Rheumatism
41 Eagle Street
London WC1

The British Rheumatism and Arthritis Association
6 Grosvenor Crescent
London SW1

The Disabled Living Foundation
346 Kensington High Street
London W14

Equipment for the Disabled
Oxford Area Health Authority
Nuffield Orthopaedic Centre
Oxford

USA

Arthritis Foundation
3400 Peachtree Road, N.E.
Atlanta, GA 30326

Arthritis Information Clearinghouse
PO Box 34427
Bethesda
Maryland 20034

National Institute of Health
Bldg 10, Room 1A05
9000 Rockville Pike
Bethesda Maryland 20205

CANADA

The Arthritis Society
920 Yonge St
Suite 420
Toronto
Ontario M4W 3J7

The Society has Division Offices in Vancouver, Calgary, Regina, Winnipeg, Montreal, Fredericton, Halifax, Charlottetown and St John's.

AUSTRALIA

Arthritis and Rheumatism Council
Wynyard House
291 George Street
Sydney
New South Wales 2000

The Australian Arthritis and Rheumatism Foundation
Chairman: Dr S. C. Milazzo
The Queen Elizabeth Hospital
Woodville
South Australia 5011

Canberra Arthritis and Rheumatism Association
PO Box 352
Woden
Australian Capital Territory 2606

The Queensland Arthritis and Rheumatism Foundation
884 Stanley Street
East Brisbane
Queensland 4169

Rheumatism and Arthritis Association of Victoria
Action House
Yarra Boulevard
Kew
Victoria 3101

The Rheumatism and Arthritis Foundation of Tasmania
84 Hampden Road
Battery Point
Tasmania 7000

The South Australian Arthritis and Rheumatism Foundation
24 King William Road
North Adelaide
South Australia 5006

The Western Australia Arthritis and Rheumatism Foundation
PO Box 7157
Cloisters Square
Perth
Western Australia 6000

NEW ZEALAND
The Arthritis and Rheumatism Foundation of New Zealand
PO Box 10–020
Southern Cross Building
Brandon Street
Wellington

SOUTH AFRICA
South Africa Rheumatism and Arthritis Association
Namaqua House
36 Burg Street
Capetown 8001

ACKNOWLEDGEMENTS

The publishers would like to thank the following people for their help and advice:
  Miss McCarroll and Mrs Lucy Benson from the physiotherapy department at the St John and St Elizabeth hospital;
  Alison Beenham, Occupational Therapist;
  The physiotherapy department of the Westminster Hospital for their help with the hydrotherapy pictures;
  Mr F. Naylor of the Disabled Drivers Association;
  Vass Anderson, Lucy Benson, Audrey Kirby and Harry Parkinson who modelled for the studio photographs.

The diagrams were drawn by Lydia Malim. The studio photographs were taken by Bill Ling and other photographs were kindly supplied by:
  Dunlop Sports Company Ltd (page 17);
  Gruner und Jahr, Munich (page 108);
  Frank Gyenes (photograph on page 56, which shows students in a planning seminar at the School of the Environment, Polytechnic of Central London);
  Brian Hale (pages 25, 29, 62, 111 and 112);
  D. G. Hodge and Son Ltd, Middlesex (page 107);
  Miller Services, Toronto (page 65);
  Galen Rowell, California (page 18);
  Phil Sheldon (page 19);
  Douglas Wilson, Washington (pages 12 and 60).

The following kindly lent equipment for use in the photographs:
  John Bell and Croyden Ltd (electric heating pad);
  The British Rheumatism and Arthritis Association;
  Doherty Medical Ltd (book rest and tilting table);
  Hag UK Ltd (chair);
  Homecraft Supplies Ltd, London (many of the gadgets in chapter six);
  Staples Ltd (bed).

INDEX

Other books in the Positive Health Guide Series

MIGRAINE AND HEADACHES   Dr Marcia Wilkinson
Understanding, controlling and avoiding the pain

HIGH BLOOD PRESSURE   Dr Eoin O'Brien and Professor Kevin O'Malley
What it means for you, and how to control it

THE HIGH-FIBRE COOKBOOK   Pamela Westland
Recipes for good health

THE DIABETICS' DIET BOOK
Dr Jim Mann

THE BACK – RELIEF FROM PAIN   Dr Alan Stoddard
Patterns of back pain – how to deal with and avoid them

PSORIASIS   Prof Ronald Marks
A guide to one of the commonest skin diseases

DIABETES   Dr Jim Anderson
A practical new guide to healthy living

STRESS AND RELAXATION   Jane Madders
Self-help ways to cope with stress and relieve nervous tension, ulcers, insomnia, migraine and high blood pressure

BEAT HEART DISEASE   Dr Risteard Mulcahy
A cardiologist explains how you can help your heart and enjoy a healthier life.

ASTHMA AND HAY FEVER   Dr Allan Knight
How to relieve wheezing and sneezing

VARICOSE VEINS   Prof Harold Ellis
How they are treated, and what you can do to help

GET A BETTER NIGHT'S SLEEP
Prof Ian Oswald and Dr Kristine Adam

ECZEMA AND DERMATITIS   Prof Rona MacKie
How to cope with inflamed skin

DON'T FORGET FIBRE IN YOUR DIET   Dr Denis Burkitt
To help avoid many of our commonest diseases

ENJOY SEX IN THE MIDDLE YEARS
Dr Christine Sandford

ANXIETY AND DEPRESSION   Professor Robert Priest
A practical guide to recovery

ACNE: HOW TO CLEAR YOUR OWN SKIN
Prof Ronald Marks

CONQUERING PAIN   Dr Sampson Lipton
How to overcome the discomfort of arthritis, backache, migraine, heart disease, childbirth, period pain and many other common conditions.

EYES: THEIR PROBLEMS AND TREATMENTS
Michael Glasspool, FRCS

OVERCOMING DYSLEXIA   Dr Bevé Hornsby

Coming soon:

THE DIABETICS' GET FIT BOOK   Jacki Winter
Introduced by Dr Barbara Boucher

THE DIABETICS' COOKBOOK
Dr Jim Mann and Roberta Longstaff